MRCPCH Part 2:
Questions and Answers for the
New Format Exam

Commissioning Editor: Ellen Green, Pauline Graham
Development Editor: Hannah Kenner
Project Manager: Andrew Palfreyman
Designer: Erik Bigland

MRCPCH Part 2: Questions and Answers for the New Format Exam

Kate H. Creese MB BCh DCH DRCOG MRCPCH
Specialist Registrar in Paediatrics
Department of Paediatrics
University Hospital of Wales
Cardiff, UK

Colin V.E. Powell MBChB DCH MRCP FRACP FRCPCH MD
Consultant Paediatrician
Department of General Paediatrics
Children's Hospital of Wales
Cardiff, UK

Patrick H.T. Cartlidge DM FRCP FRCPCH
Senior Lecturer in Child Health and Honorary Consultant Paediatrician
Department of Child Health
University Hospital of Wales
Cardiff, UK

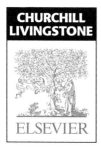

CHURCHILL
LIVINGSTONE

ELSEVIER

Edinburgh London New York Oxford Philadelphia St Louis Sydney Toronto 2008

CHURCHILL LIVINGSTONE
ELSEVIER

CHURCHILL LIVINGSTONE An imprint of Elsevier Limited

© 2008, Elsevier Limited. All rights reserved.

First published 2008

ISBN: 978-0-443-10166-3

British Library Cataloguing in Publication Data
A catalogue record for this book is available from the British Library

Library of Congress Cataloging in Publication Data
A catalog record for this book is available from the Library of Congress

Notice
Knowledge and best practice in this field are constantly changing. As new research and experience broaden our knowledge, changes in practice, treatment and drug therapy may become necessary or appropriate. Readers are advised to check the most current information provided (i) on procedures featured or (ii) by the manufacturer of each product to be administered, to verify the recommended dose or formula, the method and duration of administration, and contraindications. It is the responsibility of the practitioner, relying on their own experience and knowledge of the patient, to make diagnoses, to determine dosages and the best treatment for each individual patient, and to take all appropriate safety precautions. To the fullest extent of the law, neither the Publisher nor the Authors assume any liability for any injury and/or damage to persons or property arising out or related to any use of the material contained in this book.

The Publisher

Printed in China

Contents

Chapter 1

A male infant was born at 28 weeks' gestation weighing 940 g. He was ventilated for 16 days because of respiratory distress syndrome. He is now 25 days old and has been stable since extubation. He is in air and on full enteral feeds with a preterm neonatal formula.

You are asked to see him because he has developed an increased respiratory rate and intermittent self-limiting apnoeas.

On examination his temperature is 37.9°C, heart rate 192 bpm and respiratory rate 78 breaths/min. He has cold hands and feet and a capillary refill time of 3 s over the sternum. He has good chest movement and mild sub-costal recession. Air entry is good and his chest is clear. The heart sounds are normal but he has a 2/6 short systolic murmur at the left sternal edge. The abdomen is distended and the bowel sounds are not heard. The liver is palpable 1 cm below the costal margin; there is no other organomegaly.

a. What three investigations would you initially carry out?
   SELECT THE *THREE* MOST APPROPRIATE ANSWERS
   i. CXR
   ii. Blood culture
   iii. Lumbar puncture
   iv. AXR
   v. Cranial ultrasound scan
   vi. FBC
   vii. Echocardiogram
   viii. ECG
   ix. Coagulation screen

b. What is the most likely diagnosis?
   SELECT *ONE* ANSWER ONLY
   i. Group B streptococcal sepsis
   ii. Fungal sepsis
   iii. Pulmonary hypertension
   iv. Necrotising enterocolitis (NEC)
   v. Meningitis
   vi. Pneumonia
   vii. Intraventricular haemorrhage

Questions and Answers for the New Format Exam

ANSWERS TO CASE 1.1

a. ii. Blood culture
   iv. AXR
   vi. FBC
b. iv. Necrotising enterocolitis (NEC)

This picture in a premature neonate could be any systemic sepsis but NEC is the most likely. Initial investigations should include an AXR, FBC, and blood culture. Other investigations indicated would be serum U&E, blood glucose and blood gas. A CRP may be helpful. AXR may show intramural gas, gas in the portal vein, free gas, dilated or thickened bowel loops and a FBC may show thrombocytopaenia and/or neutropaenia.

Management in this case involves oxygen, a bolus of 20 ml/kg albumin or 0.9% sodium chloride, stopping enteral feeds and commencing i.v. maintenance fluids. Broad-spectrum antibiotics, e.g. cefotaxime and metronidazole, according to local protocol, should also be given.

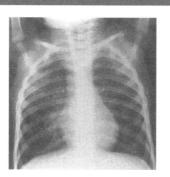

Fig 1.2

A 3-year-old girl presents with a fever 2 weeks after a 3-months stay with relatives in Africa. She is not eating and has lost weight. She has developed a cough. On examination she is pyrexial, has generalised lymphadenopathy and a palpable spleen. The CXR is shown (see Fig. 1.2).

Blood tests show:
    Hb11.3 g/dl
    WCC 12.4 × 10⁹/l
    Platelets 244 × 10⁹/l
    Malaria slide negative

a. What are the main differential diagnoses to consider?
    SELECT *TWO* ANSWERS ONLY
   i. α1-antitrypsin deficiency
  ii. Wegener's granulomatosis
 iii. Lyme disease
  iv. Miliary tuberculosis
   v. Lymphoma
  vi. Kawasaki disease

b. What investigations could help to confirm the diagnosis?
    SELECT *TWO* ANSWERS ONLY
   i. Blood culture
  ii. ELISA for *B. burgdorferi* antibodies
 iii. Bone marrow
  iv. CT chest
   v. Mantoux/Heaf test
  vi. Urinalysis

ANSWERS TO CASE 1.2

a. iv. Miliary tuberculosis (TB)
   v. Lymphoma
b. iii. Bone marrow
   v. Mantoux/Heaf test

The X-ray shows typical features of miliary TB: widespread lung infiltrates, giving a 'snowstorm' appearance. Other features suggesting miliary TB but not shown on this CXR are hilar lymphadenopathy and lobar infiltrates.

Although the history and examination are suggestive of lymphoma, the CXR does not show the expected bilateral hilar lymphadenopathy. Neither TB nor lymphomas would show diagnostic changes on blood count. Malaria cannot be excluded on a single thick and thin film, at least three should be performed if there is a real clinical suspicion.

TB can be suspected with a positive Mantoux/Heaf test in the absence of BCG vaccination, but may be falsely negative. Sputum and gastric aspirate cultures for mycobacteria may also be falsely negative, and a result can take up to 6 weeks. Biopsy of the liver or bone marrow with appropriate staining can often yield an early diagnosis. Similarly, the histology of biopsied lymph nodes would confirm a diagnosis of lymphoma.

In this case, the patient had a weakly positive Mantoux, and responded dramatically to anti-tuberculous therapy, making a biopsy unnecessary. Mycobacterium tuberculosis was cultured from gastric aspirates and full sensitivities were obtained 5 weeks after therapy was commenced.

CASE 1.3

A baby boy was admitted to the neonatal unit because of prematurity (35 weeks' gestation) and low birth weight (1700 g). He was commenced on nasogastric formula feeds which were gradually increased in volume to 150 ml/kg per 24 h by day 4. He remained alert and active and was tolerating feeds well without any vomiting but was noted to have lost more than 10% of birth weight so his feeds were increased to 200 ml/kg per 24 h by day 6. At the age of 8 days, he had lost 20% of birth weight and appeared dehydrated. A blood gas taken at this point showed:

pH 7.07
pCO_2 2.18 kPa
Base excess −25 mmol/l
Blood glucose 63 mmol/l

What is the most likely diagnosis?

SELECT *ONE* ANSWER ONLY
  i. Neonatal diabetes mellitus
 ii. Transient neonatal insulin resistance
iii. Medium chain acyl Co-A dehydrogenase deficiency
 iv. Insulinoma
  v. Congenital pancreatic agenesis
 vi. Fatty acid oxidation defect

ANSWER TO CASE 1.3

i. Neonatal diabetes mellitus

This baby has neonatal diabetes mellitus. This is a rare condition with an incidence of approximately 1 in 400 000 in the UK. Babies present with intrauterine growth retardation, followed by severe failure to thrive, hyperglycaemia and dehydration within the first 6 weeks of life.

In most babies the condition is transient and resolves at a median age of 3 months; however, they are at a higher risk of type II diabetes later in life. An abnormality of chromosome 6 can be identified in most familial cases and in 70% of sporadic cases. Many of the sporadic cases are due to paternal uniparental disomy of chromosome 6 (i.e. both inherited from the father) or due to duplication of part of chromosome 6q. Identification of the child's genotype can now help predict whether the diabetes will be permanent.

CASE 1.4

A female infant was born at term by normal delivery following a pregnancy that was uneventful apart from an influenza-like illness 2 weeks prior to delivery. She became unwell soon after delivery. Persistent pulmonary hypertension of the newborn was diagnosed and she was treated with high-frequency ventilation and nitric oxide therapy. She responded well and was extubated after 5 days. She commenced enteral feeds on the 4th day of life and achieved full feeds on day 9. She was noted to have progressive jaundice from the 10th day onwards. Other examination findings included a large broad forehead, a straight pointed nose, deep-set eyes, a soft systolic murmur, and hepato-splenomegaly.

a. What is the probable diagnosis?
   SELECT *ONE* ANSWER ONLY
   i. α1-antitrypsin deficiency
   ii. Alagille syndrome
   iii. Biliary atresia
   iv. Wilson's disease
   v. Neonatal cholestasis
   vi. DiGeorge syndrome

b. What deficiency is this child at risk of and how would you prevent it?
   SELECT *ONE* ANSWER ONLY
   i. T cells
   ii. Chymotrypsin
   iii. Folate
   iv. Fat-soluble vitamins
   v. IgG
   vi. Iron

ANSWERS TO CASE 1.4

a. ii. Alagille syndrome
b. iv. Fat-soluble vitamins

Four major categories of differential diagnosis are suggested by the initial history:
1. congenital viral infection
2. bacterial sepsis, e.g. group B streptococcal infection
3. inherited metabolic disorders, e.g. galactosaemia
4. biliary obstructive disorders, e.g. biliary atresia – extrahepatic and intrahepatic (e.g. Alagille syndrome)

However, the dysmorphic features suggest Alagille syndrome. Information about stool and urine colour would be helpful, and total and direct serum bilirubin concentration should be checked. A liver biopsy showing bile duct hypoplasia would help confirm the diagnosis and other investigations would need to be done to look for associated conditions:
- echocardiography (pulmonary stenosis/septal defect)
- radiographs of the vertebrae (vertebral anomaly)
- eye examination (posterior embryotoxin and optic nerve drusen)
- DNA analysis (JAG1 gene mutation)

Fat malabsorption secondary to chronic cholestasis is associated with a risk of fat-soluble vitamin deficiency (A, D, E, K). Fat-soluble vitamin supplementation, semi-elemental milk formula and MCT supplementation are required. Neurological sequelae of vitamin E deficiency may occur despite treatment.

Alagille syndrome (arteriohepatic dysplasia) is a dominantly inherited disorder characterised by paucity of intra-hepatic bile ducts, with resultant liver disease, along with cardiac, skeletal and ocular abnormalities and characteristic facial features. Approximately 70% of patients have mutations of Jagged 1 (JAG 1) gene (mapped to 20p12). Mortality is variable; most die of liver disease, heart disease or infections. An estimated 50% of patients require transplantation by the age of 19, due to cirrhosis, pruritus or osteodystrophy. There is an increased risk of malignancy in patients with Alagille syndrome and cirrhosis.

Physical signs may include:
- growth retardation (proportionate short stature)
- prominent forehead/frontal bossing
- deep set eyes
- hypertelorism
- posterior embryotoxon in the anterior chamber of the eye
- prominent nasal bridge
- peripheral pulmonary stenosis
- signs of hepatic dysfunction, e.g. jaundice and scratch marks from pruritus
- vertebral arch defects (hemivertebrae, butterfly vertebrae)
- rib anomalies
- hypogonadism

Associations include:
- renal anomalies
- hypoglycaemia
- mild mental retardation in about 15% of cases
- pancreatic insufficiency

CASE 1.5

A term infant was born by normal vaginal delivery with an Apgar score of 6 at 1 min and 9 at 5 min. After 10 min, he was noted to be dusky and floppy. His arterial gas showed pH 7.14, pCO_2 10.3 kPa, pO_2 2.4 kPa, and BE -6.2. He was ventilated and treated for sepsis. He required pressures of 14/4, rate of 20/min and FiO_2 of 0.21. He was still ventilated 6 days later. Three attempts at extubation failed. He also showed frequent dysrhythmias in the form of bradycardia on the ECG monitor. On examination, he was active and moving all limbs normally.

a. What is the most likely diagnosis?
   SELECT *ONE* ANSWER ONLY
   i. Hypoxic ischaemic encephalopathy
   ii. Laryngomalacia
   iii. Overwhelming sepsis
   iv. Congenital heart disease
   v. Congenital central hypoventilation syndrome

b. What are the investigations for this diagnosis?
   SELECT *THREE* ANSWERS ONLY
   i. Echocardiogram
   ii. Muscle biopsy
   iii. CSF analysis
   iv. Creatinine kinase
   v. Lung biopsy
   vi. MRI brain
   vii. CXR
   viii. FBC

ANSWERS TO CASE 1.5

a. v. Congenital central hypoventilation syndrome
b. ii. Muscle biopsy
   vi. MRI brain
   vii. CXR

The most likely diagnosis is congenital central hypoventilation syndrome. Causes include myopathies, myasthenia gravis, diaphragmatic dysfunction, a structural hind-brain or brainstem abnormality and Moebius syndrome.

Investigations include a muscle biopsy, a CXR, fluoroscopy of the diaphragm, 24-h continuous ECG monitoring, and MRI of the brain and brainstem.

Management involves careful observation of the infant's tidal volume and respiratory frequency responses to the endogenous challenges of hypercarbia and hypoxaemia, both whilst awake and during sleep. The distinction between the need for artificial ventilatory support only during sleep, or while awake and asleep, should be made after several detailed evaluations.

Following confirmation of the diagnosis, an experienced paediatric otolaryngologist should perform a tracheostomy. A transition to a home mechanical ventilator should be made whilst the child is an inpatient to allow ample time for parental training before discharge.

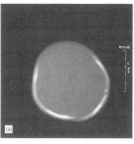 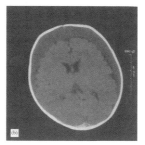 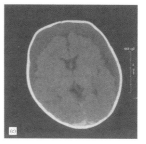

Fig 1.6

A 13-week-old infant presents because his mother noticed that his head had become larger. His head circumference had crossed from the 75th centile to the 99.6th centile over the previous 4 weeks. His fontanelle was widely open and full, but otherwise he was well and there was no history of trauma. The cranial CT scans are shown.

What do the CT scans show?

SELECT *TWO* ANSWERS ONLY
  i. Cerebral atrophy
 ii. Left posterior fracture
iii. Bilateral subdural collections
 iv. Post-haemorrhagic ventricular dilatation
  v. Cerebral oedema
 vi. Bilateral extradural collections

ii. Left posterior fracture

iii. Bilateral subdural collections

The CT scans show bilateral hypodense subdural collections overlying both cerebral hemispheres. Posteriorly, there is fresh subdural blood extending to the right. There is also a left posterior fracture; this is widened and the anterior aspect has a sclerotic margin suggesting a degree of healing. The appearance of the scan suggests haemorrhages of two different ages.

A full clinical history and examination should be taken, and a skeletal survey, bone scan, FBC and coagulation profile, metabolic screen for glutaric aciduria, and ophthalmological consultation should be arranged. A referral to social services needs to be made.

This child would need admission, consultation with the neurosurgical team, and the consultant paediatrician on duty and/or the consultant responsible for child protection must be informed, as well as the trust officer for child protection. Social services need to be contacted in order to initiate enquiry and family assessment. The general practitioner needs to be informed, and a case conference needs to be organised. The CT scan showed two haemorrhages of different ages along with the skull fracture which was starting to heal. The most likely diagnosis is child abuse. Sequelae of shaking an infant include intracranial trauma which may be life threatening, retinal haemorrhage, limb and rib fractures. A skeletal survey may include X-rays, a radioisotope bone scan and a CT brain scan if indicated, and may reveal fractures of varying ages. Other explanations should be sought, such as accidental trauma, a coagulopathy or glutaric aciduria type 1, which can be associated with subdural haemorrhages. Child protection investigation should be initiated. A doctor with expertise in child protection should undertake the latter in conjunction with social services.

CASE 1.7

A 16-year-old boy was referred by his GP with atypical absence seizures. A cranial CT scan showed multiple areas of intracranial calcification. He had been well controlled on vigabatrin for 6 years. Over the last 2 years, he had had increasing difficulty with concentration, literacy and numeracy skills, requiring considerable support.

Investigations were as follows:
    Woods light examination normal
    Renal ultrasound scan normal
    Echocardiogram normal
    Ophthalmology assessment visual field loss, visual acuity satisfactory.

What is the most likely diagnosis?

SELECT *ONE* ANSWER ONLY
    i. CMV infection
    ii. Tuberose sclerosis complex (TSC)
    iii. Congenital toxoplasmosis infection
    iv. Rett's syndrome
    v. West syndrome

ANSWER TO CASE 1.7

ii. Tuberous sclerosis complex (TSC)

TSC is a multisystem disorder affecting between 1:5000 and 1:10000 newborns. It can present at any age from the antenatal period into adulthood, with considerable variation in severity. It results from a mutation on chromosome 9 or chromosome 16. Although the condition is autosomal dominant, 60-70% of cases are sporadic and represent new mutations.

Seizures occur in 65% of patients with TSC, often presenting in infancy as infantile spasms. Seizure control can be difficult. The complete remission of fits is less common with TSC than with idiopathic epilepsy. Vigabatrin may cause visual field defects, although current evidence suggests that it is beneficial in the initial management of infantile spasms or uncontrolled epilepsy. Developmental delay occurs in up to 60% of children, learning difficulties being greatest in those presenting with infantile spasms. Control of the epilepsy may help with attention as well as psychiatric and behavioural difficulties. Children are also at increased risk of developing a subependymal giant cell astrocytoma★ (5%) in late childhood. Calcified subependymal nodules★ are found in 80% of cases of TSC. Cardiac rhabdomyomas★ are common in neonates but rarely cause complications. These decrease in mass after birth. Arterial aneurysms can also occur. Skin lesions consist of facial angiofibromas★, periungal fibromas★, shagreen patch★, fibrous plaque on the forehead★ and hypomelanic (ash leaf) macules★.

Renal complications include angiomyolipomas★ (80%), polycystic kidney disease (20%) and renal cell carcinoma (1%). Pulmonary lymphangioleiomyomatosis★ is rare and occurs exclusively in females, usually presenting in adulthood with respiratory impairment.

★A definitive diagnosis of TSC requires two of these major features.

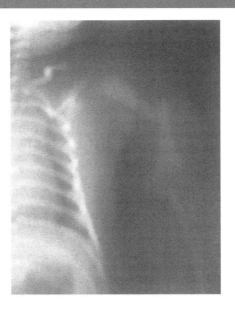

Fig 1.8

This is an X-ray of a term baby taken at 1 h of age. The birthweight was 4495 g.

What should be specifically checked on initial examination?

SELECT *ONE* ANSWER ONLY
  i. Presence of a distal pulse
  ii. Associated fracture of the clavicle
  iii. Associated nerve injury (palsy)
  iv. Blood sugar
  v. Moro reflex

ANSWER TO CASE 1.8

i. Presence of a distal pulse

The X-ray shows a mid-shaft spiral fracture of the left humerus with around 60° of angulation. This was sustained during delivery (shoulder dystocia). Limitation of passive motion due to pain and crepitance will be present. The examination should include an assessment of motor function and a check for the presence of a distal (radial) pulse. This injury can be associated with radial nerve injury leading to wrist drop and inability to extend the fingers at the metacarpophalangeal joints. The differential diagnosis will include brachial plexus injury or fracture of the clavicle. The former will present as either Erb's, Klumpke's or Erb–Duchenne–Klumpke palsy.

Management involves ensuring adequate analgesia and supporting the affected arm, for example with the use of a net bandage against the chest wall to immobilize in flexion at the elbow.

The fracture is likely to unite within 2 weeks despite the angulation without any operative intervention and the long-term outlook is good. Angular deformities will be spontaneously corrected with growth.

CASE 1.9

A 7-year-old girl presented with a 2-month history of unexplained episodes of pyrexia. In that period she had also developed widespread lymphadenopathy and had had one nose bleed which had stopped spontaneously. On examination she was pale with palpable lymph nodes in the cervical, pre-auricular and inguinal regions. She also had an enlarged liver and spleen. A peripheral blood count and film showed:

Hb 7.4 g/dl
WCC 6.3 × 10^9/l
Neutrophils 0.5 × 10^9/l
Platelets 91 × 10^9/l
Blasts 20%

a. What is the most likely diagnosis?
SELECT *ONE* ANSWER ONLY
  i. Aplastic anaemia
  ii. Non-Hodgkin's lymphoma
  iii. Acute lymphoblastic leukaemia
  iv. Fanconi's anaemia
  v. Acute myeloid leukaemia

b. What features of this condition signify a favourable prognosis?
SELECT *TWO* ANSWERS ONLY
  i. Age >1 year
  ii. Male sex
  iii. High white count
  iv. Age <10 years
  v. Low white count

ANSWERS TO CASE 1.9

a. iii. Acute lymphoblastic leukaemia
b. i. Age >1 year
   v. Low white count

The likely diagnosis in this girl is acute lymphoblastic leukaemia. Features that signify a favourable prognosis include age >1 year and under 10 years, female sex and a low white count.

Patients with high white counts and, therefore, large tumour mass are at risk of tumour lysis syndrome once chemotherapy starts. To minimise the effects of large quantities of intracellular ions (such as uric acid and phosphate) being deposited in the kidneys and causing renal failure, patients should receive hydration ($3\,l/m^2/24\,h$) and allopurinol for approximately 12 h before treatment starts.

1. Staphylococcal scalded skin syndrome
2. Rubella
3. Measles
4. Kawasaki disease
5. Impetigo
6. Scarlet fever
7. Infectious mononucleosis
8. Still's disease
9. Roseola infantum
10. Erythema infectiosum

For each of the following case scenarios select the most likely diagnosis from the list above.

a. A 5-year-old boy has a bright red, punctate erythematous rash which blanches on pressure. It seemed to begin in the axillae associated with some perioral pallor and relative facial sparing. The skin feels like 'sandpaper'. The rash fades and desquamation occurs on the hands and feet. A thick white exudate develops on the tongue which peels leaving a bright red 'raspberry tongue' with prominent papillae.

b. A salmon-coloured, reticulate macular rash develops mainly over the extensor surfaces of the limbs in a 5-year-old boy with a swinging temperature; he is also complaining of hot, swollen, painful knees and left elbow and on examination is found to have a palpable spleen. Investigations reveal an ESR of 95, although the FBC, CRP and CXR are normal.

c. A 4-year-old girl presents to her general practitioner with a 1-day history of a high fever, associated with the appearance of a discrete, maculopapular rash, which was first noted on the face and neck. She had been unwell for 3-4 days previously with upper respiratory tract symptoms and conjunctivitis.

ANSWERS TO CASE 1.10

a. 6. Scarlet fever

Scarlet fever occurs when the infectious organism (usually a group A streptococcus) produces erythrogenic toxin in an individual who does not possess neutralizing anti-toxin antibodies. The incubation period is 2-4 days following a streptococcal infection, usually in the pharynx. The rash, initially on the neck, appears around day 2, and quickly becomes punctate and generalised. It is prominent in the flexures, but typically spares the face, palms and soles. The rash lasts about 5 days, and is followed by desquamation of the skin. The face may be flushed but characteristically with circumoral pallor. Early in the disease the tongue has a white coating through which prominent bright red papillae can be seen ('strawberry tongue'), but this coating later disappears, leaving a raw-looking red colour ('raspberry tongue'). Complications include peritonsillar or retropharyngeal abscesses and otitis media.

b. 8. Still's disease (systemic onset juvenile chronic arthritis)

Still's is the commonest type of juvenile chronic arthritis (about 70% of cases), and is divided into 3 types (systemic, pauci- or oligoarticular and polyarticular). Systemic is usually seen in children of under 5 years of age. Presenting features include a high fever, a characteristic rash with patches of erythema, often appearing in the evening and exacerbated by warmth, and lymphadenopathy, splenomegaly and pericarditis. Arthritis or arthralgia may not be present initially, but may develop later in the course of the disease.

c. 3. Measles

Measles is a highly communicable disease spread by droplets, and remains one of the commonest childhood infections in developing countries. The incubation period varies from 8 to 14 days. There are two distinct phases of illness: the pre-eruptive catarrhal stage, followed by the exanthematous stage. Initial symptoms include cough, coryza and conjunctivitis for 2-4 days, followed by fever and the appearance of a discrete, then a confluent, red, maculopapular rash. It typically first appears behind the ears and then sequentially on the face, neck, trunk, upper limbs, then buttocks and lower limbs. Koplik spots (white spots on a red buccal mucosa) are found 1-2 days before the rash and last 3-5 days. Measles is infectious from 1 to 2 days before the onset of symptoms to 4 days after the appearance of the rash. Complications include otitis media, pneumonia and encephalitis.

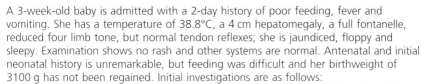
A 3-week-old baby is admitted with a 2-day history of poor feeding, fever and vomiting. She has a temperature of 38.8°C, a 4 cm hepatomegaly, a full fontanelle, reduced four limb tone, but normal tendon reflexes; she is jaundiced, floppy and sleepy. Examination shows no rash and other systems are normal. Antenatal and initial neonatal history is unremarkable, but feeding was difficult and her birthweight of 3100 g has not been regained. Initial investigations are as follows:

- Haematology: Hb 13.2 g/dl, WCC 22.7 × 10^9/l, Platelets 32 × 10^9/l, Prothrombin time 23 s, APTT 78 s
- Biochemistry: Na 127 mmol/l, K 4.7 mmol/l, urea 6.8 mmol/l, creatinine 52 μmol/l, CRP 198 mg/l, glucose 1.2 mmol/l, ALT 256 IU/l, albumin 28 g/l, bilirubin 249 μmol/l (conjugated 26%), venous pH 7.26, bicarbonate 16 mmol/l, ammonia 52 mmol/l, lactate 1.9 mmol/l
- Microbiology: blood culture, no growth at 48 h. CSF microscopy: Gram-negative bacilli, polymorphs +++ (confirmed on culture), urine leucocytes ++, coliforms >10^5 organisms/ml
- Radiology: CXR normal

After the baby's hypoglycaemia has been corrected, she is started on i.v. cefotaxime and ampicillin, and nasogastric tube feeds, but 8 days later there is little discernable improvement. The repeat CSF culture is sterile, and although she has been apyrexial since treatment day 4, she continues to be drowsy, jaundiced and to vomit. A CT brain scan is normal. Further test results:

- Haematology: Hb13.6 g/dl, WCC 12.7 10^9/l, Platelets 47 × 10^9/l, Prothrombin time 25 s, APTT 77 s
- Biochemistry: Na 129 mmol/l, K 3.2 mmol/l, urea 7.1 mmol/l, creatinine 51 μmol/l, CRP 65 mg/l, glucose 2.3 mmol/l, alanine aminotransferase 397 IU/l, albumin 25 g/l, bilirubin 312 μmol/l (conjugated 26%)
- Urine: sterile, Clinistix protein +, bilirubin +, pH 5, glucose -, Clinitest +

What is the most likely underlying diagnosis?

SELECT *ONE* ANSWER ONLY
  i. alpha-1-antitrypsin deficiency
  ii. Galactosaemia
  iii. Biliary atresia
  iv. Alagille syndrome
  v. Pseudo-Bartter syndrome
  vi. Neonatal amyloidosis
  vii. Herpes simplex infection
  viii. Wilson's disease

ANSWER TO CASE 1.11

ii. Galactosaemia

Galactosaemia is the most likely diagnosis in this case and an assay of galactose-1-phosphate uridyl transferase (Gal-1-P UT) should be requested to confirm it.

Management involves stopping milk feeds and starting a galactose-free formula. In a neonate with a fever, a full septic screen is mandatory. Neonatal sepsis with *Escherichia coli* should always prompt a consideration of galactosaemia as an underlying diagnosis. Further clues in this case are acidosis; hypoglycaemia; the presence of hepatomegaly with deranged liver function and coagulopathy; and acidic urine that contains reducing substances other than glucose. The condition presents only once feeding has been commenced and the lactose in breast or standard formula milk is metabolised to glucose and galactose. The consequent accumulation of galactose-1phosphate (in the absence of Gal-1-P UT) is injurious to the parenchymal cells of the liver, kidney and brain. Clinistix tests only for the presence of glucose so a positive Clinitest but negative Clinistix result indicates the presence of a reducing susbstance other than glucose (galactose). Stopping milk feeds and starting a galactose-free formula usually results in a dramatic improvement. Early diagnosis by Gal-1-P UT assay and dietary restriction of lactose intake do not prevent long-term complications, which include neuro-developmental problems, particularly with language acquisition, and premature ovarian failure with infertility in females. The endogenous production of galactose may be responsible for these long-term effects. Follow-up throughout life is mandatory.

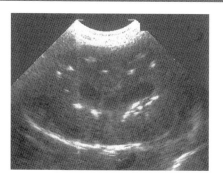

Fig 1.12

An infant born at 33 weeks' gestation with a birthweight of 1596 g (3rd–10th centile) and a head circumference of 26.6 cm (3rd centile), was, at delivery, in good condition, but had bilateral arthrogryposis with fixed flexion deformities of arms, bilateral talipes and fixed flexion of both hips. He made few spontaneous movements and at 6 h of age generalized seizures began, which were difficult to control despite anticonvulsant medication. An initial FBC showed:

Hb 13.8 g/dl
Platelets $56 \times 10^9/l$
Total WCC $4.64 \times 10^9/l$
Neutrophil count $1.54 \times 10^9/l$
Lymphocytes $2.56 \times 10^9/l$
Nucleated red cell count 51 per 100 WBC

A cranial ultrasound scan was also performed which is shown in Figure 1.12.

a. What is the most likely diagnosis?
SELECT *ONE* ANSWER ONLY
 i. Arthrogryposis multiplex congenita
 ii. Infant of a drug-abusing mother
 iii. GM1 gangliosidosis
 iv. Congenital CMV infection
 v. Congenital rubella infection

b. What investigations would you perform to confirm the diagnosis?
SELECT *THREE* ANSWERS ONLY
 i. Serology for congenital infections
 ii. CSF for CMV
 iii. Urine toxicology
 iv. Hearing test
 v. Ophthalmology review
 vi. Skull X-ray
 vii. Genetic testing

c. What does the ultrasound scan show?
SELECT *ONE* ANSWER ONLY
 i. Arteriolar calcification
 ii. Subependymal calcification
 iii. Periventricular leukomalacia
 iv. Intraventricular haemorrhages with dilatation
 v. Periventricular parenchymal echodensities

ANSWERS TO CASE 1.12

a. iv. Congenital CMV infection
b. i. Serology for congenital infections
   ii. CSF for CMV
    v. Ophthalmology review
c. v. Periventricular parenchymal echodensities

The most likely diagnosis is congenital CMV infection. To confirm the diagnosis, urine must be sent for CMV culture, and serology for congenital viral infections. PCR for CMV can be performed on urine, serum and CSF. Examination of the retina is important to look for evidence of chorioretinitis.

The USS shows bilateral periventricular parenchymal echodensities, indicating areas of periventricular haemorrhage, infarction or possibly calcification. The lack of shadow behind the echodensities is against them being calcified lesions but this is better confirmed with CT scanning. Maternal serology and serum PCR for congenital viral infections will help confirm the diagnosis. Serology can also be checked from booking bloods.

Congenital CMV is the commonest cause of congenital infection with an estimated frequency of 0.3-0.4% in the UK. However, over 90% of infants with congenital CMV are asymptomatic in the neonatal period, although many are growth retarded. Previous infection is very common with 50% of women seropositive at booking. The risk of fetal infection depends on whether infection is primary or a re-activation. There is a 25% risk of transplacental transmission with primary infection and a 2% risk during re-activation. However, because so many women are seropositive at conception, reactivation produces many more cases. The risk of sequelae also varies depending on whether infection is primary or a re-activation. Most infants who are asymptomatic in the neonatal period develop normally and have a normal IQ, and this includes most of those infected by re-activation. In one study following primary infection, 33% of infants had sequelae; however, following re-activation, only 14% had sequelae, and these tended to be less severe. Mortality from symptomatic neonatal CMV infection is between 10 and 30%.

Important sequelae include sensorineural deafness, microcephaly, developmental delay and cerebral palsy.

An 8-year-old boy from a travelling family presented to the emergency department with a fever of 39.5°C and a painful swollen right ankle. He had been coryzal over the previous 3 days. There was a history of a fall 2 weeks previously but he had fully recovered. There was no other significant past medical history. He did not receive any of his childhood immunisations. The family is currently living on a site near a local moor. On examination, there was no cardiovascular compromise. He had a coryza with associated cervical lymphadenopathy. His right ankle was hot and swollen, and he resisted any attempt to move it. Remaining examination was unremarkable. The following results were obtained:

Hameoglobin 9.4 g/dl
MCV 69.7 fl
WBC 20.9 × 10^9/l
Neutrophils 16.2 × 10^9/l
Platelets 525 × 10^9/l
CRP 118 mg/dl (normal range <10 mg/dl)

The decision was made to start intravenous benzylpenicillin and flucloxacillin. As these were being administered the nurse noticed a purpuric rash that had not been there previously.

What is the most likely diagnosis?

SELECT *ONE* ANSWER ONLY

i. Meningococcal septic arthritis
ii. Henoch–Schönlein purpura
iii. Von Willebrands disease with intraarticular haematoma
iv. Lyme disease
v. Disseminated intravascular coagulation
vi. Parvovirus B19 infection

ANSWER TO CASE 1.13

i. Meningococcal septic arthritis

The specific treatment is high-dose intravenous third-generation cephalosporin anti-biotics. Supportive treatment is critical to survival in meningococcal septicaemia, and these children often require invasive monitoring and treatment in intensive care. Contact tracing with appropriate antibiotic prophylaxis and immunisation of at-risk individuals in the immediate community is normally performed by public health physicians. Definitive diagnosis in suspected septic arthritis is made following analysis of aspirate from the affected joint. Performed under surgical conditions, this also gives the opportunity to wash out the joint and immobilise in a functional position. The co-existence of arthritis and a purpuric rash is classically seen in Henoch–Schönlein purpura (HSP) which is the most common of the vasculitides affecting children. Septic arthritis with DIC should be considered. The most common organisms isolated in septic arthritis are *Staphylococcus aureus*, *Streptococcus pneumoniae* and *Salmonella sp.*, and in the unim-munised child *Haemophilus influenzae b* and *Neisseria meningitidis* are well recognised but rare causes. Mycobacteria may also cause septic arthritis but this is less commonly associated with DIC. Lyme disease (*Borrelia burgdorferi*) is frequently associated with an arthropathy. It is caused by the bacterium carried by ticks in endemic areas (often open moorland in the UK). There is usually a history of flu-like symptoms, and patients may have a rash with purpuric elements, although this usually evolves from the classic rash of erythema migrans. Both purpura and arthritis are recognized as manifestations of Parvovirus B19 infection or Fifth disease, although the laboratory results in this case are more in keeping with a bacterial aetiology.

A 12-year-old West Indian boy presented with symmetrical swelling of his fingers. One week previously, he had complained of a severe sore throat and had developed a papular rash after having been prescribed amoxicillin. The hand swelling had developed gradually during the day of presentation. On examination, he was afebrile. There was widespread lymphadenopathy and mild pharyngitis. There was left upper quadrant tenderness and his spleen was palpable 3 cm below the costal margin. On examination of both hands he complained of pain over the metacarpophalangeal and phalangeal joints. Both ankles were swollen. He had restricted movement in all affected joints.

What is the most likely diagnosis?

SELECT *ONE* ANSWER ONLY
   i. Coxsackie infection
  ii. Epstein–Barr virus infection
 iii. Lyme disease
  iv. Thalassaemia
   v. Sickle cell syndrome
  vi. Post-streptococcal arthritis
 vii. Juvenile idiopathic arthritis

ANSWER TO CASE 1.14

ii. EBV infection

The most likely diagnosis is EBV infection. The physical findings are consistent with this diagnosis. Arthritis and arthralgias are common in many viral infections. Joint lesions are due to the deposition of immune complexes and not direct viral infection. The arthritis is usually transient and self-limiting. The prodrome in this case included a papular rash following amoxicillin as classically seen in EBV. Investigations should include blood film, Hb electrophoresis, viral serology, complement, and streptococcal serology. A blood film may be diagnostic in a sickle cell crisis. It may also show characteristic lymphocyte morphology in EBV infection. Hb electrophoresis will diagnose sickle cell disease. A request for viral serology should include EBV, hepatitis A and B, CMV, coxsackie, echovirus and adenovirus. A stool sample for virology may increase the chances of viral identification. Rubella should be considered in unimmunised individuals. Complement C3 and C4 will be reduced in systemic lupus erythematosus as well as post-streptococcal arthritis. An elevated or rising ASOT titre indicates recent streptococcal infection but may take a week or more to rise.

Positive serology confirmed EBV infection. Dactylitis is frequently the presenting complaint in sickle cell disease which must be excluded in a boy of West Indian origin. Post-streptococcal arthritis may exist as a distinct disease entity or be part of rheumatic fever. JIA and systemic lupus erythematosus need to be considered as part of the initial differential diagnosis.

CASE 1.15

An infant born at 28 weeks' gestation suddenly collapses at 3 weeks of age. She was initially ventilated for 10 days and has since been stable on NCPAP in 26% O$_2$. She is currently receiving total parenteral nutrition via a percutaneous long line situated in the right atrium and is on 4 ml/h of enteral feed via a nasogastric tube. At the time of collapse, she is poorly perfused with a capillary refill time of 6 s, is tachycardic at 195/min, and has a blood pressure of 36/28 mmHg. There is no heart murmur but heart sounds are quiet. An arterial gas reveals a mixed respiratory and metabolic acidosis. Following ventilation and stabilisation, a CXR shows a massively enlarged cardiac shadow with normal lung fields. Her cranial ultrasound shows bilateral grade 1 intraventricular haemorrhage.

What is the most likely diagnosis?

SELECT *ONE* ANSWER ONLY

  i. Cardiac tamponade
  ii. Tension pneumothorax
  iii. Overwhelming sepsis
  iv. Congenital heart disease
  v. Increased intracranial pressure
  vi. An inborn error of metabolism

ANSWER TO CASE 1.15

i. Cardiac tamponade

Differential diagnosis should include cardiac tamponade, septicaemia, congenital heart disease, or an inborn error of metabolism. Echocardiography is the investigation of choice, which will not only confirm a pericardial effusion, but also exclude congenital heart disease.

Cardiac tamponade in this case has occurred secondary to a long line which has migrated into the pericardial sac. Percutaneous long lines should be positioned just outside the heart either in the superior or inferior vena cava. It is vital that the tip is clearly visualised. If it is placed in the right atrium, it must be withdrawn and re-X-rayed. If the tip cannot be seen, contrast medium should be used.

Management involves removal of the long line and drainage of the pericardial effusion using the subxiphisternal approach. After cleaning the skin, a 22/24 G cannula should be inserted at an angle of 30° to the skin, directed towards the left shoulder. Aspirated fluid should be sent for microbiological and biochemical assay. Only if the effusion reaccumulates will it be necessary to leave a catheter in situ. In this case, the drained fluid was confirmed to be TPN.

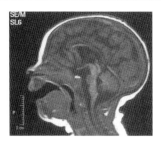

Fig 1.16.A

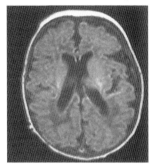

Fig 1.16.B

Following induction of labour at 41 weeks' gestation for maternal hypertension, an infant (birth weight 3000 g) was delivered normally and cried immediately, requiring no resuscitation. At approximately 8 h of age, after transfer to the post-natal ward with her mother, she was admitted to the neonatal unit because of tachypnoea, poor feeding and jitteriness. The blood glucose, electrolytes and serum creatinine were normal. A septic screen was performed and she was commenced on i.v. antibiotics. A blood gas on admission to the neonatal unit showed:

pH 7.323
pCO_2 2.81 kPa
Bicarbonate 11.2 mmol/l
Base excess −11.9 mmol/l
Lactate 7.50 mmol/l (<2 mmol/l)

Other investigations showed:
CSF clear/colourless with no organisms or white blood cells
Glucose 3.5 mmol/l
Lactate 16.2 mmol/l.

The results of an MRI brain scan are shown above.

a. What do the results indicate?
   SELECT *ONE* ANSWER ONLY
   i. Compensated respiratory acidosis
   ii. Metabolic acidosis
   iii. Mixed metabolic and respiratory acidosis
   iv. Compensated metabolic acidosis
   v. Respiratory alkalosis

b. What other investigations are necessary?
   SELECT *THREE* ANSWERS ONLY
   i. Skin biopsy
   ii. Urine amino acids
   iii. DNA analysis
   iv. Plasma ammonia
   v. Serum organic acids
   vi. Electroencephalogram

c. What is the differential diagnosis?
   SELECT *THREE* ANSWERS ONLY
   i. Methylmalonicacidaemia
   ii. Glycogen storage disease type 1
   iii. Organic acid disorders
   iv. Urea cycle disorders
   v. Pyruvate dehydrogenase deficiency
   vi. Non-ketotic hyperglycinaemia

ANSWERS TO CASE 1.16

a. iv. Compensated metabolic acidosis
b. i. Skin biopsy
   ii. Urine amino acids
   iv. Plasma ammonia
c. ii. Glycogen storage disease type 1
   iii. Organic acid disorders
   v. Pyruvate dehydrogenase deficiency

The results show a primary lactic acidosis with a cerebral lactic acidosis. She is blowing off her CO_2 to compensate for the acidosis.

The MRI scan shows dilated lateral ventricles and a thin corpus callosum. Investigations should include urinary amino and organic acids, serum amino acids and plasma ammonia. Skin biopsy may be helpful for fibroblast culture and specific cytogenetic analysis. Differential diagnosis of primary lactic acidosis includes glycogen storage disease type I, organic acid disorders, disorders of pyruvate metabolism, disorders of gluconeogenesis and electron transport chain defects.

This infant presented with non-specific features but the initial blood gas found a severe lactic acidosis. There was no evidence of an earlier hypoxic ischaemic insult therefore a lactic acidosis secondary to a hypoxic event was extremely unlikely. The MRI scan suggests an early antenatal insult and these changes are common in infants with primary lactic acidosis. Lactic acidosis presents a difficult diagnostic problem as primary lactic acidosis produces many of the circulatory problems which cause secondary lactic acidosis. It is important in this situation to seek the advice of a biochemist or clinician with expertise in metabolic diseases, as investigation and therapy can be difficult. Some conditions require treatment with carbohydrate supplementation and others are made worse by this regimen. This infant had pyruvate dehydrogenase deficiency which has an incidence of 1 in 200000 and is usually inherited as an X-linked dominant condition. It typically presents with severe acidosis or profound neurological deficit and structural brain lesions. It is usually caused by deficiency of the E1α-subunit which is on the short arm of the X chromosome. Both hemizygous males and heterozygous females are affected, nearly all cases being due to new mutations. Patients with structural brain lesions are usually females with severe enzyme lesions which destroy patches of the brain in which the mutant gene is active. Males usually present with early severe acidosis.

CASE 1.17.1

A 3-year-old boy is admitted to hospital following two episodes of abnormal movements. His mother reported that on two consecutive mornings, whilst having his breakfast, the right side of his face and his right hand were twitching for about 30 s. He appeared to be conscious throughout both episodes. Afterwards, he recovered completely, although following the second episode he fell asleep on the sofa. His twin brother used to have uncomplicated febrile convulsions in the past. He and his brother were adopted at birth. Growth parameters are all on the 50th centile. Clinical examination including fundoscopy was entirely normal. EEG showed left-sided centrotemporal spikes.

What is the most likely diagnosis?

SELECT *ONE* ANSWER ONLY
   i. Temporal lobe epilepsy
  ii. Hypnagogic myoclonic seizures
 iii. Febrile convulsion
  iv. Simple partial seizures
   v. Benign Rolandic epilepsy
  vi. Complex partial seizures

ANSWER TO CASE 1.17

v. Benign Rolandic epilepsy

In all cases of seizures, a detailed developmental history should be taken. The family history should also be taken, although this is more difficult in this case since the child was adopted.

Differential diagnosis from the history and examination includes benign Rolandic epilepsy of childhood or simple partial seizures. The EEG here showed left-sided centro-temporal spikes, which is typical for benign Rolandic epilepsy of childhood and can also be bilateral. A sleep EEG often intensifies the spike activity. Further investigations like neuro-imaging are not indicated because of the diagnostic nature of the EEG and the absence of any neurological abnormalities on clinical examination.

The best treatment for benign Rolandic epilepsy is not to treat! The condition is benign and because the seizures usually occur during sleep or on waking, it is well tolerated. If the seizures are interfering with schooling or quality of life, carbamazepine or valproate may be used. The age of onset is between 3 and 13 years. Prognosis is excellent. Seizures commonly stop at the age of 12 years and the EEG normalizes several years later. There is no increased risk of seizure development in later life. This is a genetic disorder transmitted as an autosomal dominant trait. Forty percent of close relatives have a history of febrile convulsions or epilepsy.

An 8-month-old infant has frequent episodes of hypoxia post-operatively following uncomplicated bilateral inguinal herniotomies. He is now 12 h post-operation and his oxygen saturation is 88% in air. He has required bag and mask ventilation on a couple of occasions for apparent apnoeas. On examination, he is extremely pale and tachycardic with a heart rate of 190/min. His heart sounds are normal, but he has a gallop rhythm. He is tachypnoeic with a respiratory rate of 60/min and has mild intercostal recession, but his chest is entirely clear. He has a palpable liver 2 cm below the costal margin. He has bilateral haematomas at the incision sites. He is well grown for his age, but his mother mentions that he always looks a bit pale. His post-operative Hb is 4 g/dl and his platelet count is 224×10^9/L. His activated partial thromboplastin time was very prolonged with a normal thrombin and prothrombin time.

What is the likely underlying condition?

SELECT *ONE* ANSWER ONLY

  i. Bernard–Soulier syndrome
 ii. Antithrombin III deficiency
iii. Cardiomyopathy
 iv. Vitamin K deficiency
  v. Haemophilia A
 vi. Von Willebrand's disease

ANSWER TO CASE 1.18

v. Haemophilia A

The most likely diagnosis here is haemophilia A (although haemophilia B cannot be excluded).

This little boy had developed heart failure secondary to anaemia. Because of the extensive haematomas, it is important to ask whether he has a history of easy bruising and nose bleeds and if there is a family history of bleeding disorders. Particular attention should be paid to any history of prolonged bleeding following simple procedures such as circumcision and childbirth.

Investigations should include a repeat FBC and film, coagulation profile and CXR. The blood film will look at red blood cell morphology. In this patient, the anaemia was normocytic. A preoperative Hb had not been done. A clotting profile is warranted in any patient with unexplained/disproportionate bruising, particularly if male. His activated partial thromboplastin time was very prolonged with a normal thrombin and prothrombin time. A CXR will exclude causes for his respiratory deterioration other than heart failure. This patient did have haemophilia A as confirmed by measuring his clotting factors. He had a very low level of factor VIII (2.5%). A level of <1% is consistent with severe haemophilia and usually presents with easy bruising in infancy. They do not bleed excessively from cuts or from mucosal surfaces unless raw areas exist.

Treatment involves a blood transfusion and an injection of factor VIII concentrate. The circulating level was raised by 30%, which usually achieves haemostasis, using 15 units/kg of factor VIII.

Haemophilia A is inherited as an X-linked recessive condition and parents need genetic counselling for future pregnancies.

CASE 1.19

A term baby boy was admitted to the neonatal unit at 4 h of age with grunting and respiratory distress. On admission he was noted to be micrognathic, with a cleft palate, syndactyly of the 2nd and 3rd toes of both feet and mildly reduced tone.

a. What is the most likely cause of his respiratory distress?
SELECT *ONE* ANSWER ONLY
  i. Respiratory distress syndrome
  ii. Sepsis
  iii. Micrognathia
  iv. Congenital heart disease
  v. Hypotonia

b. What would your initial management be?
SELECT THE *TWO* MOST APPROPRIATE ANSWERS
  i. Nasopharyngeal airway care
  ii. Place him supine
  iii. CPAP
  iv. Intubate and ventilate
  v. Septic screen and treat empirically with antibiotics

Progress was slow and he remained reluctant to feed, requiring top-ups via a naso-gastric tube to ensure adequate calorie intake. At 4 weeks of age he developed persistent vomiting. A repeat septic screen was performed. The venous blood gas revealed a pH of 7.49, bicarbonate of 36.2 mmol/l and potassium of 3.0 mmol/l.

c. What syndrome is he most likely to have?
SELECT *ONE* ANSWER ONLY
  i. Holt–Oram
  ii. Pierre–Robin
  iii. Smith–Lemli–Opitz
  iv. Ellis–Van Creveld
  v. Rubinstein–Taybi

ANSWERS TO CASE 1.19

a. iii. Micrognathia
b. i. Nasopharygeal airway
   v. Septic screen and treat empirically with antbiotics
c. iii. Smith–Lemli–Opitz

His respiratory distress is secondary to his micrognathia and cleft palate (the Pierre–Robin syndrome), causing soft-tissue obstruction of his airway by his posteriorly placed tongue. His hypotonia will contribute to worsen this effect. Sepsis as a cause for respiratory distress must be considered in all neonates irrespective of gestation and this may coincide with structural abnormalities.

Management of his respiratory distress involves the following: a prone position, a nasopharyngeal airway to help with breathing, and a maxillofacial team and speech therapy opinion regarding the fitting of a plate over the cleft to aid feeding and feeding advice. A septic screen including CXR should be considered in all unwell neonates.

This baby developed hypertrophic pyloric stenosis (obstruction to the outflow tract of the stomach secondary to muscle hypertrophy). A test feed can be performed to confirm this diagnosis, palpating an olive-shaped mass in the right hypochondrium. If the test feed is equivocal then an ultrasound scan is helpful.

This baby was subsequently diagnosed as having Smith–Lemli–Opitz syndrome, a disorder of cholesterol synthesis which is associated with an increased rate of pyloric stenosis. The main features of this syndrome are developmental delay, poor growth, cleft palate, genital anomalies and syndactyly or polydactyly.

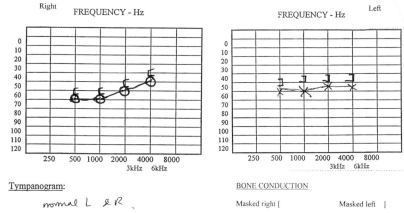

Right   FREQUENCY - Hz

FREQUENCY - Hz   Left

Tympanogram:

normal L & R

BONE CONDUCTION

Masked right [Masked left]

Fig 1.20

What does this pure tone audiogram show and what might cause this picture?

SELECT THE *BEST PAIR* OF ANSWERS

A. Right conductive hearing loss
B. Bilateral moderate conductive hearing loss
C. Bilateral mixed conductive and sensori-neural hearing loss
D. Within normal limits
E. Bilateral moderate sensori-neural hearing loss
F. Right sensorineural hearing loss
G. Bilateral high-frequency sensori-neural hearing loss

1. Pendred syndrome
2. Intrauterine group B strep infection
3. Recurrent secretory otitis media
4. Neonatal conjugated hyperbilirubinaemia
5. Upper respiratory tract infection
6. Bilateral perforated ear drums
7. Bilateral cleft palate

ANSWER TO CASE 1.20

E. and 1.
(Bilateral moderate sensori-neural hearing loss and Pendred syndrome)

Subjects with normal hearing can hear pure tones 20 dB (decibel hearing loss) or less. The air conduction thresholds in the right ear (circle) show a hearing level of 60 dB at 500 Hz–1000 Hz, rising to 40 dB at 4000 Hz. On the left (cross) the range is 50-55 dB. There is equal impairment of air and bone conduction in sensorineural hearing loss. In conductive hearing loss there is a difference of at least 15 dB between air and bone conduction ('air-bone gap').

Causes of sensori-neural hearing loss may be congenital or acquired.

Congenital causes of sensori-neural hearing loss

Isolated sensorineural hearing loss is the commonest cause of sensori-neural deafness (inheritance autosomal recessive but autosomal dominant and sex-linked transmission also occurs). Severe (65-80 dB) and profound (85 dB) sensorineural loss affects 1 in 1000 children, but the incidence can be as high as 1 in 40 in very low birth weight, ventilated babies.

Syndromes with deafness are much less common, and include:
- Chromosomal, e.g. Turner's syndrome
- Ophthalmological, e.g. Usher's (with progressive retinitis pigmentosa and cataracts)
- Ectodermal/pigmentary, e.g. Waardenburg's (autosomal dominant, dysmorphic features such as broad nasal root, hyperplasia of medial aspect of eyebrows, white or grey lock of hair or early greying, heterochromia of irises)
- Skeletal/craniofacial, e.g. Treacher–Collins (autosomal dominant, hypoplasia of mandible, high-arched or cleft palate, oblique palpebral fissures, microtia with absent external auditory canal). Goldenhar's syndrome also features ear abnormalities with deafness, and vertebral anomalies, eye defects (coloboma, cataracts or epibulbar dermoids) and characteristic facies of frontal bossing, small mandible and nostrils.
- Metabolic/endocrine/renal, e.g. Pendred syndrome (hypothyroidism), Alports (renal), Jervell–Nielson (prolonged QT interval).

Acquired causes of sensorineural deafness

- Intrauterine infection (CMV, rubella, toxoplasmosis, syphilis)
- Perinatal asphyxia
- Neonatal hyperbilirubinaemia
- Infections, e.g. bacterial meningitis (pneumococcus, *H. influenzae*, and meningococcus)
- Drugs, e.g. aminoglycosides

Chapter 2

CASE 2.1

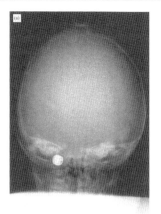 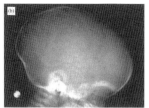

Fig 2.1

A 13-week-old baby girl is referred to the outpatient department for a prominent and protruding forehead. According to her mother this has always been the case though to a lesser extent than when she was born. The child is otherwise well, weight following the 0.4th centile, length along the 9th centile and head circumference on the 50th centile. The parents are not concerned about the head shape but the child's GP is and hence the referral.

On examination the child appears well. She has a very small anterior fontanelle and frontal prominence.

What do the skull X-rays show?

SELECT *TWO* ANSWERS ONLY

  i. Wormian bones
 ii. Ridging of sutures
 iii. Fused sagittal suture
 iv. Fused lamboid suture
  v. Dolicocephalic head shape
 vi. Fused coronal suture

iii. Fused sagittal suture
v. Dolicocephalic head shape

Both X-ray views show a fused sagittal suture throughout its length. The dolicocephalic head shape is seen in Figure 2.1.1.

The diagnosis here is sagittal craniosynostosis. Other features to look at in the examination include head shape, e.g. long and narrow – dolicocephalic, short and square – brachycephalic; ridging of sutures; and fingers and toes should be examined for abnormalities.

Treatment involves urgent referral to a designated centre for craniofacial surgical assessment. A multidisciplinary team comprising the neurosurgeon, plastic surgeon and neurologist manage the condition.

Craniosynostosis occurs when there is lack of dural growth from restricted cranial expansion or limited brain growth. The most common cause of isolated craniosynostosis is constraint of the fetal head. The incidence of this problem is about 1 in 1000 births.

Sagittal craniosynostosis is the most common type, with a 3:1 predilection for males, due to more rapid head growth in males during late gestation. The head shape is dolicocephalic. Coronal craniosynostosis may occur by itself, or as part of an autosomal dominant disorder such as Crouzon syndrome, Apert syndrome, Pfeiffer syndrome, or Saethre-Chotzen syndrome, in which various types of limb abnormalities may be present. Lambdoid craniosynostosis accounts for less than 3% of all cases.

The designated centres for craniosynostosis treatment in the UK are in Oxford, Birmingham, and Great Ormond Street.

CASE 2.2

A male infant was born at 31 weeks by caesarean section for reduced fetal movements and being small for gestational age. He developed severe respiratory distress requiring intermittent ventilation for 2 months. At birth, he was noted to have a spreading petechial rash. He then developed a persistent conjugated hyperbilirubinaemia. He also had grade 3 intraventricular haemorrhage, dilated ventricles and intracranial parenchymal calcification. He developed grade 3 retinopathy of prematurity and bilateral chorioretinitis. CMV PCR was highly positive, and blood cultures were negative. The infant received a 3 month course of ganciclovir, with a fall in his PCR value. He currently has hepatosplenomegaly and microcephaly with global developmental delay.

a. What could be the causes of the severe respiratory distress?
SELECT THE *TWO* MOST APPROPRIATE ANSWERS
  i. HIE
  ii. CCAML
  iii. Central hypoventilation syndrome
  iv. CMV pneumonitis
  v. Surfactant deficient lung disease
  vi. Bilateral pleural effusions

b. What could be the cause of the hyperbilirubinaemia?
SELECT THE *MOST APPROPRIATE* ANSWER
  i. Total parenteral nutrition
  ii. Intrahepatic calcification
  iii. CMV hepatitis
  iv. Haemolysis
  v. Physiological jaundice

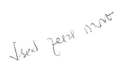

ANSWERS TO CASE 2.2

a. iv. CMV pneumonitis
   v. Surfactant deficient lung disease
b. iii. CMV hepatitis

Congenital CMV infection affects approximately 1% of newborn infants, although most are asymptomatic. CMV is a herpes virus. It can be transmitted in utero (with a vertical transmission rate of 40%), perinatally from infected cervical secretions or postnatally, acquired from breast milk or through blood transfusion. CMV is excreted in saliva, urine, semen, cervical secretions, stool and tears. Approximately 90% of infants are clinically asymptomatic and have a favourable outcome, although they are at risk (5-17%) of developing sensorineural hearing loss, chorioretinitis, learning difficulty and neurological deficits. About 10% exhibit a wide variety of signs and symptoms such as intrauterine growth retardation, jaundice, hepatosplenomegaly, petechiae or purpura, thrombocytopenia, pneumonia, chorioretinitis (10-20% of symptomatic infants), intra-cranial calcification (often periventricular, affecting 25-50% of symptomatic infants), sensorineural hearing loss (50%), seizures and microcephaly. Of those infants who are asymptomatic, 90% have long-term sequelae such as sensorineural hearing loss (usually in first 3 years of life), motor and intellectual disability, seizures and chorioretinitis.

The diagnosis is made by viral culture of the urine, blood, CSF or nasopharynx (in first 3 weeks of life). Other tests include enzyme linked immunosorbent assay (for CMV) specific IgM, or PCR.

Ganciclovir is currently being investigated for use in infants with symptomatic con-genital infection and CNS disease. Anecdotal evidence suggests that critically ill new-borns with CMV pneumonia may benefit from this drug.

A 10-year-old boy presented with his first afebrile convulsion. His parents describe a 5-minute generalised tonic–clonic convulsion, from which he fully recovered 90 min later. He is developmentally normal, with no previous medical history of note. He has become upset recently over his continued bed-wetting, and his GP recently prescribed a 'night-time tablet', his parents say, to help. Since starting he has been dry at night.

a. What is the likely cause of the fit?
   SELECT *ONE* ANSWER ONLY
   i. Pseudoseizures
   ii. Dehydration
   iii. Epilepsy
   iv. Hyponatraemia
   v. Benign Rolandic seizures
   vi. Hypernatraemia

Oxybutinin

b. What investigation should be done first?
   SELECT *ONE* ANSWER ONLY
   i. Serum electrolytes
   ii. Water deprivation test
   iii. EEG
   iv. Lumbar puncture
   v. ECG

c. What is the treatment?
   SELECT *TWO* ANSWERS ONLY
   i. i.v. fluid bolus of 0.9% saline
   ii. Stop the medication
   iii. Restriction of his fluid intake
   iv. Sodium valproate
   v. Carbamazepine
   vi. No treatment necessary

ANSWERS TO CASE 2.3

a. iv. Hyponatraemia
b. i. Serum electrolytes
c. ii. Stop the medication
    iii. Restriction of fluid intake

This seizure is secondary to hyponatraemia with water overload, secondary to medication. He had been prescribed 'desmotabs' (vasopressin) 3 weeks earlier to control his enuresis. The risk is from water overload, and the information sheet provided with desmotabs, stresses the importance of avoiding excessive evening drinking. As with any medicine, there is always a risk of overdose, intentional or accidental.

It is imperative to measure serum electrolytes, which would demonstrate low sodium. Water restriction is usually sufficient to correct hyponatraemia if the cause is water overload, especially in this case when the source of the water overload is removed (i.e. stop the medication). Regular checking of the serum electrolytes confirms the normalisation of the sodium.

Rarely hyponatraemia must be treated more rapidly, i.e. if the patient continues to fit. In this case, where there is water overload, infusing a small volume of hypertonic saline helps shift fluid from the intracellular to the vascular space, and the extra water is excreted by the kidneys.

CASE 2.4

A 3-week-old boy was admitted with pyrexia, irritability, poor feeding and a high-pitched cry. He had been born by spontaneous vaginal delivery at 41 weeks' gestation, weighing 3600 g. On examination his temperature was 38.8°C, there were two small pustules on his chest; he disliked any handling and showed neck retraction. He was tachycardic but well perfused.

Investigation results included:
CSF microscopy:
    RBC 220/mm^3
    WCC 80/mm^3 (90% lymphocytes)
    No organisms
CSF glucose 3.2 mmol/l
CSF protein 1.2 g/l
Blood glucose 4.4 mmol/l

6 h after admission, he started to have focal, right-sided seizures.

a. What is the most likely diagnosis?
    SELECT *ONE* ANSWER ONLY
  i. Staphylococcal scalded skin syndrome
  ii. Impetigo
  iii. Tuberculous meningitis
  iv. Herpes encephalitis
  v. Meningococcal meningitis
  vi. Non-accidental injury

b. What treatment should be commenced?
    SELECT *TWO* ANSWERS ONLY
  i. i.v. fluid bolus
  ii. i.v. antibiotics and acyclovir
  iii. i.v. mannitol
  iv. Steroids
  v. Anticonvulsants

ANSWERS TO CASE 2.4

a. iv. Herpes encephalitis
b. ii. i.v. antibiotics and acyclovir
   v. Anticonvulsants

Diagnoses of viral encephalitis, bacterial meningitis and sepsis elsewhere should all be considered. A full septic screen should be performed.

Treatment should include acyclovir and antibiotics, and anticonvulsants for seizure control. The CSF findings are more suggestive of viral infection but antibiotics should be continued until cultures are negative. The vesicle fluid can be examined by electron microscopy for herpes virus particles.

Neonatal herpes simplex infection may occur in disseminated form, localized (skin, eye, mouth), or with an encephalitis. It is usually caused by HSV type 2. In 50% of cases of herpes simplex encephalitis no vesicles appear. Neonatal herpes encephalitis has a mortality of 15% and a high risk of long-term neurological sequelae (>50%).

CASE 2.5

A term male infant was admitted to the neonatal intensive care unit at 12 h of age because he was cyanosed. His apgar scores were 9 at 1 min and 9 at 5 min. He had fed well though the midwife had felt he had never been pink.

His oxygen saturation was 68% in air and 70% in 3 l of oxygen via nasal prongs. The saturation remained low despite increasing supplemental oxygen and he developed increasing respiratory distress. On examination his respiratory rate was 64 breaths/min and heart rate 180 bpm. Chest examination revealed clear lung fields. He had an easily palpable cardiac pulsation, normal peripheral pulses, normal heart sounds and no audible murmur. The rest of the examination was unremarkable. His CXR showed a slightly large heart with normal lung fields.

a. What is the most likely diagnosis?
   SELECT *ONE* ANSWER ONLY
   i. Transposition of the great arteries
   ii. Tricuspid atresia with VSD
   iii. Truncus arteriosus
   iv. Total anomalous pulmonary venous drainage
   v. Pulmonary atresia
   vi. Fallot's tetralogy

An intravenous treatment was commenced on the baby.

b. What are the complications of this treatment?
   SELECT *THREE* ANSWERS ONLY
   i. Seizures
   ii. Hypokalaemia
   iii. Apnoea
   iv. Hypertension
   v. Hypotension
   vi. Arrhthymias
   vii. Haemorrhage
   viii. Hyperkalaemia

ANSWERS TO CASE 2.5

a. i. Transposition of the great arteries
b. ii. Hypokalaemia
    iii. Apnoea
    v. Hypotension

Transposition of the great arteries is the most common cyanotic congenital heart disease (CCHD) accounting for approximately 5% of all congenital heart disease. It often co-exists with other cardiac defects, e.g. VSD that allow for better mixing of blood.

The closing of the ductus arteriosus results in loss of mixing if there is no or only a small VSD, so it is crucial to commence an infusion of prostaglandin as quickly as possible, to maintain patency of the ductus arteriosus.

However, this treatment is not without problems, so, where possible, should be administered in an intensive care setting. Apnoeas can lead to the baby requiring ventilation, especially if transfer to a specialist cardiac centre is needed. Other side-effects of prostaglandin include fever, flushing, hypotension and hypokalaemia.

Definitive treatment for transposition is changing. Until the mid-1990s, a balloon atrial septostomy was performed early on; then a permanent procedure was carried out at 6-9 months (Mustard or Senning operations). Now many centres maintain the duct by the prostaglandin infusion and a definitive repair (arterial switch) is carried out within the first few days of life.

CASE 2.6

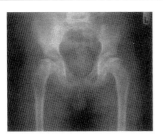

Fig 2.6.A

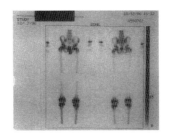

Fig 2.6.B

An 8-year-old, previously healthy boy, presented with a 6 h history of fever, irritability and drowsiness. On admission he was febrile, and had a widespread petechial rash. A diagnosis of meningococcal septicaemia was suspected. Blood cultures were taken, and he was commenced on intravenous antibiotics and resuscitated with 4.5% human albumin solution. He deteriorated and was transferred to ITU where he was ventilated. He required infusions of dobutamine, adrenaline and noradrenaline to maintain his blood pressure, and he developed severe adult respiratory distress syndrome. He then developed acute tubular necrosis and was haemofiltered. He had numerous vasculitic lesions on his skin. Other complications were a pneumothorax, pneumomediastinum and pulmonary haemorrhage. Both hips were normal at the onset of his illness. His length of stay on ITU was 6 weeks but eventually he appeared to make a full recovery.

At outpatient review 4 months later, he complained of pain on walking and back pain, and had limited abduction of both hips. His plain X-ray and bone scan are shown.

What is the most likely cause of his symptoms?

SELECT *ONE* ANSWER ONLY

  i. Osteoporosis
 ii. Avascular necrosis
iii. Renal osteodystrophy
 iv. Cerebrovascular event
  v. Systemic lupus erythematosus
 vi. Systemic juvenile arthritis

ANSWER TO CASE 2.6

ii. Avascular necrosis

The plain X-ray shows severe flattening and sclerosis of both femoral heads. The bone scan shows reduced uptake of the tracer indicating avascular necrosis of both hips. Sequelae of meningococcal meningitis are commonly neurological, notably deafness. Complications arising from meningococcal septicaemia include the problems of the vasculitic skin lesions and gangrene. Bony lesions are less commonly described. The most likely aetiology of the avascular necrosis in this case is ischaemia either secondary to embolism or hypoperfusion. The presence of bilateral femoral intravenous and intra-arterial lines may have contributed towards the vascular compromise. It is possible that with more aggressive therapy and improved survival with severe meningococcal septi-caemia, long-term complications such as avascular necrosis will become more evident necessitating long-term follow-up.

CASE 2.7

A 1-year-old child was referred by her GP to the community paediatric team, the main parental concern being delayed motor milestones. The child was unable to sit or weight-bear, but her speech development was normal. Other than one lower respiratory tract infection, her past medical history was unremarkable.

On examination, she was floppy and weak. While supine, her legs flopped outwards at the hips. There was also paucity of leg movement. In ventral suspension, the child exhibited a rag-doll effect and head lag. She had muscle-wasting and tongue fasciculation. Her head circumference was on the 50th percentile and her height and weight on the 9th percentile.

a. What is the most likely diagnosis?
   SELECT *ONE* ANSWER ONLY
   i. Spinal muscular atrophy (SMA) type 2
   ii. SMA type 1
   iii. Scapulo-facial muscular dystrophy
   iv. Guillain–Barre syndrome
   v. Duchenne muscular dystrophy
   vi. Werdnig–Hoffman disease
   vii. Prader–Willi syndrome

b. What investigations would help confirm your diagnosis?
   SELECT *TWO* ANSWERS ONLY
   i. EEG
   ii. Spinal MRI
   iii. CSF protein
   iv. Survival motor neurone (SMN) gene-testing
   v. Oligoclonal bands in CSF
   vi. Muscle biopsy
   vii. Creatine phosphokinase level

ANSWERS TO CASE 2.7

a. i. Spinal muscular atrophy (SMA) type 2
b. iv. Survival motor neurone (SMN) gene-testing.
   vii. Creatine phosphokinase

The diagnosis here is SMA type 2. The differential diagnosis includes congenital myotonic dystrophy, congenital muscular dystrophy, congenital myopathy and congenital neuropathy, although the fasciculation makes them unlikely. The diagnosis can be confirmed by gene-testing for the SMN gene. Other investigations include creatine phosphokinase level, chromosome analysis, TSH titre and urine amino/organic acid concentrations.

SMA is an autosomal recessive degenerative disease of the anterior horn cells of the spinal cord with loss of motor neurones leading to muscle atrophy. Three main types exist depending on age and acuteness of presentation. Overall incidence is 1 in 6000 newborns. Usually presenting with weakness, wasting and, often, tongue fasciculation, all forms are progressive, with a shortened life expectancy due to respiratory compromise secondary to scoliosis.

SMA type 1 (also known as infantile or Werdnig–Hoffman disease) presents early; it is usually obvious by 3 months of age and rapidly progresses. Affected infants die by 3 years. Infants have floppy paralysis below neck level. Facial and bulbar muscle strength is normal. Because of the paralysis of the intercostal muscles, respiration depends on the diaphragm.

SMA type 2 presents after 3 months of age. It runs a subacute course. Age at death is widely variable, although survival into the 4th decade is recognized. Infants may appear to develop normally and even stand before regressing. The majority of children lead a wheelchair existence.

SMA type 3 (juvenile, Kugelberg–Welander) tends to present after 2 years of age with pelvic and shoulder girdle weakness after a period of normal walking.

Mutations of the SMN gene (SMN1) are known to be responsible for SMA, particularly homozygous deletion of exons 7 and 8 of the SMN1 gene on chromosome 5. This is known to occur in 98% of all cases of SMA.

Prognosis depends on the type of SMA:
    type 1 – 95% mortality by 18 months
    type 2 – 60% mortality by 10 years
    type 3 – mean age of death is 51 years

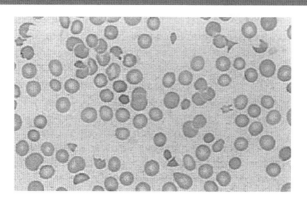

Fig 2.8

A 6-year-old girl was admitted with vomiting, abdominal pain and bloody stools. An ultrasound scan could not rule out an intussusception. After considered surgical review, she went to theatre for a laparotomy. There was no intussusception but she appeared to have large bowel colitis. She had no bowel surgery and returned to the ward. Stool culture was sent and it was considered that she probably had an infective colitis. Her FBC and U&E on admission were normal; 2 days post-operatively they showed:

Hb 9.5 g/dl
WCC 19.4 × 10^9/l
Platelets 16 × 10^9/l
ESR 2 mm/h
Na 134 mmol/l
K 4.4 mmol/l
Urea 11.8 mmol/l
Creatinine 80 μmol/l

Her urine output reduced and urinalysis showed her to have microscopic haematuria but no proteinuria. Her blood film showed haemolysis with fragmentation of red blood cells.

What is the likely diagnosis?

SELECT *ONE* ANSWER ONLY

   i. Henoch–Schonlein nephritis
  ii. Amyloidosis
 iii. Autoimmune haemolytic anaemia
  iv. Shigella nephropathy
   v. Post-infectious glomerulonephritis
  vi. Haemolytic uraemic syndrome (HUS)

ANSWER TO CASE 2.8

vi. Haemolytic uraemic syndrome (HUS)

With evidence of acute haemolysis, thrombocytopenia and deteriorating renal function, the likely diagnosis is HUS. This is associated with *Escherichia coli* 0157 (which was isolated in this case) and can occur in epidemics. HUS occurs commonly in children younger than 4 years of age and is the most frequent cause of acute renal failure in children. Diarrhoea occurs for 5-7 days before haemolysis and thrombocytopenia develop, and renal failure follows several days later.

Management involves strict attention to fluid balance, renal function (focusing on acid–base balance, hyperkalaemia and increasing creatinine), monitoring for and treating hypertension, and watching for fluid overload. As the haemolysis and anaemia deteriorate, a blood transfusion may be required and this may exacerbate fluid overload. Thus transfusion has to be carefully considered. The child may go on to require dialysis as renal function deteriorates.

There is a good prognosis with 65-85% complete recovery. There is a mortality rate of 5-10% during the acute phase of the illness, and a few patients develop end-stage renal disease.

CASE 2.9

A 12-year-old boy presented with difficulty breathing and abdominal pain. He had seen the GP twice in the past with episodes of diarrhoea which subsided spontaneously. On this occasion, the family mentioned a recent visit to a relative's wedding in central Africa but said they had sought advice regarding immunisations and took prophylaxis against malaria. On examination, he was unwell, febrile and looked pale. There was dullness and decreased breath sounds in the base of the right lung. The right upper quadrant was tender and the liver was palpable 4 cm below the costal margin.

a. What are the most likely diagnoses suggested by this history and examination?
   SELECT THE *TWO* BEST ANSWERS
   i. Right-sided pneumonia
   ii. Viral hepatitis
   iii. Malaria
   iv. Amoebic liver abscess
   v. Hydatid disease
   vi. Typhoid
   vii. Giardiasis

b. What investigations would best help confirm the diagnosis?
   SELECT *TWO* ANSWERS ONLY
   i. Blood gas
   ii. Lung function tests
   iii. CT scan
   iv. Stool for microscopy and culture
   v. Hepatitis serology
   vi. FBC and film

ANSWERS TO CASE 2.9

a. i. Right-sided pneumonia
    iv. Amoebic liver abscess
b. iii. CT scan
   iv. Stool for microscopy and culture

The findings are consistent with an amoebic liver abscess. Differentials include a pyogenic abscess and a right-sided pneumonia.

Relevant history would include change in bowel pattern, and history of diarrhoea and dysentery, particularly while in Africa. It is, however, important to remember that there is evidence of previous or concomitant dysentery in only 50% of amoebic liver abscesses.

A CXR may show a raised diaphragm. There may also be an effusion and other signs of inflammation. An abdominal USS localizes and delineates the abscess in most cases. More than 95% of liver abscesses may be detected by CT scan. A FBC will usually show leucocytosis. CRP/ESR is elevated. Serology is useful. Stools, if examined when fresh, will show signs of infection in about one-third of patients, usually amoebic cysts. Only in a minority are the amoebea demonstrable.

Metronidazole or tinidazole are the drugs of choice for the treatment of invasive amoebiasis. A luminal amoebicide is essential at the end of treatment for eradication of amoebea from the lumen of the bowel. Broad spectrum antibiotics are indicated for suspected septicaemia.

Complications include secondary bacterial infection, extension or rupture into the peritoneal cavity, pleural cavity and or lungs. Blood-borne spread may result in a brain or lung abscess.

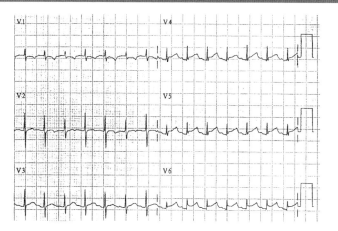

Fig 2.10

An 18-month-old girl has been treated on the children's ward for meningococcal septicaemia. This diagnosis has been assumed on the basis of a localised purpuric rash and the growth of Gram-negative cocci on blood culture. She responds well to intravenous fluids and antibiotics but after an initial recovery has developed increasing tachypnoea. One of the investigations performed was an ECG.

What abnormalities can be seen on the ECG and what is the diagnosis?

SELECT THE *BEST PAIR* OF ANSWERS

A. Low voltage QRS complexes and raised ST segments

B. Sinus tachycardia with right heart strain

C. QTc of 0.55 s

D. Right ventricular hypertrophy

E. Peaked T waves

1. Second-degree heart block

2. Cardiomyopathy

3. Pericarditis

4. Prolonged QT syndrome

5. Pulmonary hypertension

ANSWER TO CASE 2.10

A. and 3.

The ECG shows low voltage QRS complexes in all the chest leads and raised ST segments. This is consistent with diagnosis of pericarditis, a known complication of meningococcal infection. The pericardial effusion is generally purulent but may also result from an autoimmune response and this typically occurs during the recovery phase of the illness.

An emergency cardiac assessment should be obtained where possible as pericardiocentesis or surgical drainage may be required as was the case with this girl (she had a purulent effusion with tamponade). However, symptomatic management may sometimes be all that is required where the pericarditis and effusion have resulted from an immune response as these generally prove to be transient reactions.

A 4-month-old child is admitted to hospital with pyrexia and irritability. She appears unwell with decreased responsiveness and hypotonia. A septic screen is done and she is commenced on broad spectrum antibiotics. Blood, urine and CSF cultures are negative. Stool cultures grow adenovirus. Her blood film shows vacuolated lymphocytes. She recovers from the infection but on follow-up remains hypotonic with global developmental delay. Her weight is on the 50th centile and head circumference on the 90th centile. She is noted to have multiple Mongolian blue spots, coarse features, peripheral oedema and hepatosplenomegaly. The fundi appear abnormal, and after pupillary dilatation, a cherry red spot is seen at the macula.

a. What diagnoses should be considered?
   SELECT THE *THREE* BEST ANSWERS
   i. Hunter's syndrome
   ii. Tay–Sach's disease
   iii. Niemann–Pick disease
   iv. GM1 gangliosidosis
   v. Gaucher's disease
   vi. Cornelia De Lange syndrome
   vii. Pseudohypoparathyroidism

b. What other investigations may be helpful?
   SELECT THE *THREE* BEST ANSWERS
   i. CT head
   ii. Cultured skin fibroblast enzymes
   iii. Lateral spine X-rays
   iv. EEG
   v. Bone marrow examination
   vi Karyotype
   vii. Bone biochemistry

ANSWERS TO CASE 2.11

a. ii. Tay–Sach's disease
    iii. Niemann–Pick disease
    iv. GM1 gangliosidosis
b. ii. Cultured skin fibroblast enzymes
    iii. Lateral spine X-rays
    v. Bone marrow examination

With children presenting like this, it is important to seek further information from the history; such as her developmental status before presentation, and whether there was any suggestion of developmental regression. Is there any parental consanguinity or family history of note? Does she startle easily to sound?

Possible diagnoses to be considered include GMI gangliosidosis, Tay–Sach's disease, Sandhoff's disease, Hurler's syndrome, I cell disease and Niemann–Pick disease.

GM1 gangliosidosis was the diagnosis in this child. This is an autosomal recessive condition due to deficient b galactosidase. There is accumulation within neurones and viscera of compounds containing a terminal b galactosidase residue. This causes the characteristic findings of coarse features, subcutaneous oedema, hepatosplenomegaly and progressive neurological deterioration. A cherry red spot on the retina is found in 50%. The condition is associated with extensive and unusual Mongolian blue spots. Hyperacusis occurs.

White blood cell or cultured skin fibroblast enzymes are diagnostic. Lateral spine X-rays may show anterior breaking. Bone marrow examination reveals foamy cells.

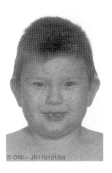
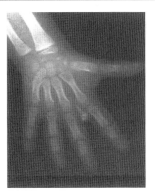

© OMI – JR110101/04

Fig 2.12

A 5-year-old boy presented with subcutaneous nodules in the right hand, right foot and right ear. The lesions between his right index and middle fingers caused him difficulty in writing. He was otherwise fit and well. He was born at 42 weeks' gestation, symmetrically growth retarded with a birth weight of 2390 g. His neonatal period was complicated by hypoglycaemia, thrombocytosis and a seizure. On examination his height was between the 50th and 75th centiles and his weight was on the 99.6th centile. He had a round face with narrow, slightly up-slanting palpable fissures. An X-ray of the right hand (see above) showed multiple soft tissue areas of calcification and ossification. The following investigations were performed:

Ca 2.44 mmol/l
Phosphate 1.35 mmol/l
ALP 566 mU/l
PTH 5.8 pmol/l (normal range 1.0-6.1 pmol/l)
TSH 2.7 mU/l (normal range 0.5-6.0 mU/l)
Thyroxine 105 nmol/l (normal range 70-180 nmol/l)

What is the most likely diagnosis?

SELECT *ONE* ANSWER ONLY

  i. Pseudohypoparathyroidism
 ii. Secondary hypoparathyroidism
iii. McCune–Albright syndrome
 iv. Secondary hyperparathyroidism
  v. Hyperparathyroidism
 vi. Pseudopseudohypoparathyroidism
vii. Albright's polyostotic fibrous dysplasia

ANSWERS TO CASE 2.12

vi. pseudopseudohypoparathyroidism

Pseudopseudohypoparathyroidism (a type of Albright hereditary osteodystrophy) is the most likely diagnosis. Confirmation can be made by sending DNA for mutational analysis of GNAS gene.

Albright hereditary osteodystrophy (AHO) is a syndrome characterized by short stature, round facies, shortened 4th and 5th metacarpals/tarsals, and subcutaneous calcification. AHO is often associated with pseudohypoparathyroidism (PHP), hypocalcaemia and elevated PTH (PHP 1A) where PTH resistance leads to hypocalcaemia. Mental retardation is present in some cases.

Patients with pseudopseudohypoparathyroidism have *normal* calcium metabolism and PTH levels with isolated AHO (phenotype).

Mutations in the GNAS1 gene which encodes the alpha subunit of the adenyl cyclase stimulating G protein (Gsα), lead to features of AHO. Managing patients with AHO involves dietary advice, identifying learning difficulties at school and regular blood tests looking for PTH resistance. In patients with PHP, hypocalcaemia is treated with vitamin D and calcium supplements aiming to suppress PTH levels into the normal range.

CASE 2.13

An infant was born following a normal vaginal delivery at term. His mother was a primigravida and was blood group O negative with no antibodies detected during pregnancy. No resuscitation was required at birth. He bottle fed normally taking adequate volumes of milk but was noted to be jaundiced at 12 h of age. The total bilirubin was 250 μmol/l, blood group A positive and direct Coombs test negative. He was commenced on phototherapy but the bilirubin continued to rise and he had an exchange transfusion at 36 h of age when the total bilirubin concentration was 400 μmol/l.

a. What is the most likely cause of the jaundice and what other investigations would help to confirm this?
   SELECT *ONE* ANSWER ONLY
   i. Alpha thalassaemia
   ii. Glucose-6-phosphate dehydrogenase deficiency
   iii. Rhesus incompatibility
   iv. ABO incompatibility
   v. Pyruvate kinase deficiency
   vi. Hereditary spherocytosis

b. What other management steps are necessary?
   SELECT *TWO* ANSWERS ONLY
   i. Screening of siblings
   ii. Iron supplementation
   iii. Folate supplementation
   iv. Careful monitoring of subsequent pregnancies because of increasing severity with each pregnancy
   v. Repeat Hb level

ANSWERS TO CASE 2.13

a. iv. ABO incompatibility
b. iii. Folate supplementation — folic acid
    v. Repeat Hb level

Other investigations to confirm the diagnosis include a blood film and Hb to look for evidence of haemolysis. Group A haemolysin assay can be performed in the mother. This test is not often performed as the diagnosis is usually obvious but if there is a doubt it can help to confirm ABO incompatibility. Other causes of haemolysis such as glucose-6-phosphate dehydrogenase deficiency and pyruvate kinase deficiency may also need to be excluded, although these do not usually cause such a rapid rise in the bilirubin in the first 24 h.

The timing of this infant's jaundice suggests a haemolytic cause. No antibodies were detected during pregnancy so Rhesus disease or haemolysis due to other transfusion related antibodies is unlikely. The direct Coombs test is also negative which is against a haemolytic cause, but the combination of Group O in the mother and Group A in the infant means that ABO incompatibility is a possibility and severe haemolysis can occur with this condition despite a negative direct Coombs test. Anaemia in this condition is usually only mild. The jaundice in ABO incompatibility is caused by A or B haemolysins which are IgG antibodies that can cross the placenta (unlike the usual A or B IgM antibodies which cannot cross the placenta). The incidence of ABO incompatibility is 1 in 150 births, but severe disease is only seen in approximately 1 in 3000. The severity of ABO incompatibility is very variable and some infants will show very little evidence of haemolysis despite a positive Coombs test, whereas other infants will show severe haemolysis and will require exchange transfusion. The Coombs test does not indicate the severity of the condition. 40-50% of cases occur in first born infants and it does not become more severe with subsequent pregnancies.

Repeat bilirubin checks are necessary until the level is under control. Folate supplementation is needed, because of continued haemolysis and follow-up to check for late anaemia (although this is much less likely to happen than with Rhesus haemolytic disease). Late anaemia is very unlikely in children with ABO incompatibility who did not require an exchange transfusion.

1. Cystic Fibrosis
2. Wiskott–Aldrich syndrome
3. Congestive cardiac failure
4. Kartagener's syndrome
5. Bartter syndrome
6. Schwachmann–Diamond syndrome
7. Fanconi syndrome
8. Diamond–Blackfan syndrome
9. Partial anomalous pulmonary venous drainage
10. Congenital cystic malformation of the lung

For each of the following case scenarios select the most likely diagnosis from the list above.

a. A 10-hour-old, male, term infant with a birth weight of 3260 g is noted to be grunting. Antenatal progress had been uneventful, although situs inversus was noted on the scans. The Apgar scores were 7 at 1 min and 10 at 5 min. No resuscitation was required. On examination his temperature was 35.8°C, heart rate 130 bpm, respiratory rate 35/min. The oxygen saturation in air was 96%. He was grunting and had a capillary refill time of 4 s. Heart sounds were normal and femoral pulses were palpable. On chest auscultation there was bilateral and equal air entry, with some intercostal recession. Blood gas was normal, and the grunting settled with warming. However, he continued to have signs of respiratory distress with tachypnoea, recession and an intermittent supplemental oxygen requirement for several weeks. The CXR revealed scattered streaky shadows in the lung fields but was otherwise normal. An ultrasound showed a structurally normal heart with a left-sided liver and aorta.

b. A 3-month-old, breast-fed boy was seen in hospital. At 4 weeks of age, he had been admitted to hospital appearing pale; he had Hb of 2.9 g/dl. He was also neutropaenic. Extensive investigation revealed only that his IgM to EBV was positive. At 3 months, he weighed 3760 g (birth weight 2960 g). His skin was dry and flaky, and his stools were loose, pale and pungent. He had received two courses of oral antibiotics from the GP for upper respiratory tract infections. CXR was normal. Sweat test results were as follows:
volume of sweat obtained – 134 mg
sweat Na – 17 mol/l
sweat Cl –14 mmol/l.

c. A 6-month-old boy was referred by the GP with a cough and weight loss. He had had a cough on and off since birth and vomiting for 2 weeks. His weight had dropped from the 50th centile at birth to below the 3rd centile. The cough sometimes produced green sputum. He was born at term and was well following birth. He was admitted at 2 months with a persistent cough and blue episodes at the end of coughing. A naso-pharyngeal aspirate was negative for respiratory syncytial virus and after 5 days, he was sent home. On examination, he was afebrile. Heart rate was 110 bpm, blood pressure 85/60 mm Hg. He was tachypnoeic, with a respiratory rate of 40/min. His oxygen saturation was 86% in air. He had intercostal recession, but a clear chest on auscultation. His skin was loose and he looked very malnourished. Initial blood results showed:
Na 120 mmol/l
Hb 11.1 g/dl
K 2.3 mmol/l
WCC 13.6 × 10⁹/l
Urea 5.8 mmol/l
Platelets 394 × 10⁹/l
Creatinine 47 µmol/l
pH 7.579
Urine Na 5 mmol/l
Bicarbonate 40.5 mmol/l.

a. 4. Kartagener's syndrome

Persistent respiratory symptoms in the neonate with no obvious cause and possible situs inversus suggest primary ciliary dyskinesia (PCD) and Kartagener's syndrome. PCD denotes all congenital abnormalities of ciliary function whereas the term Kartagener's syndrome refers to the subgroup of patients with PCD and situs inversus. Persistent moist cough or persistent and unexplained respiratory distress in the neonatal period should raise suspicion. Rhinitis or nasal congestion begins on the day of birth, persists and is difficult to treat. Although average presentation is at 16 years, nasal stuffiness and heavy sputum production may have occurred since early childhood. Impaired mucus clearance leads to severe sinopulmonary disease with chronic sinusitis, otitis media with hearing impairment, nasal polyps and bronchiectasis. Most males are infertile and females risk ectopic pregnancy. Rarer complications include hydrocephalus secondary to abnormalities of the brain ependymal cilia, complex congenital heart disease and biliary atresia. Diagnosis is by biopsy and treatment is similar to that used for cystic fibrosis.

b. 6. Schwachmann–Diamond syndrome

Schwachmann–Diamond syndrome comprises cyclical neutropaenia, recurrent pyogenic infections and pancreatic failure. 70% have thrombocytopaenia, 50% anaemia. Skin is commonly dry and flaky, and is improved by pancreatic supplementation. Sweat Na is normal. Inheritance is autosomal recessive. 25% go on to develop myelodysplastic syndrome.

c. 1. Cystic Fibrosis

The most likely diagnosis is a pseudo Bartter syndrome caused by excessive sweat electrolyte loss in undiagnosed cystic fibrosis (CF). In CF chronic sweat electrolyte loss may be aggravated by an intercurrent illness, precipitating metabolic consequences. There is a lack of adequate salt intake to counteract the loss through sweat. The biochemistry shows severe hyponatraemia, hypokalaemia and a metabolic alkalosis. The hallmark of both Bartter and pseudo-Bartter syndrome is a very low serum Na and potassium. The distinction between them is that there is no primary renal disease is pseudo-Bartter syndrome. Extensive loss of serum electrolytes causes the kidneys to try and reabsorb electrolytes in the tubules, and the loss of electrolytes activates the normal compensatory mechanisms, including the renin-angiotensin pathway. Vomiting may have exacerbated the salt loss.

A 35-year-old asymptomatic Somali refugee mother living in the UK for 4½ years is found on antenatal screening to be HBsAg positive.

Which of the following statements are true?

SELECT *THREE* ANSWERS ONLY

   i. Hepatitis screening is unreliable in HIV +ve patients

  ii. With a +ve HBe antigen, there is a 50% chance of mother-to-child transmission

 iii. If mother is +ve for HBe antigen, the baby must receive hep B vaccination and immunoglobulin at birth

 iv. If mother is +ve for HBe antibody, the baby must receive immunoglobulin at birth

  v. HBe antibody positivity confers protection against transmission to baby

 vi. Immunoglobulin must be given within 6 h of birth

vii. With no detectable HBe antibody, there is no risk of infectivity from the mother

viii. Neonatal hepatitis B vaccination is given in 2 doses

 ix. Vertical transmission can be reduced by 40% by active immunisation at birth

  x. Hepatitis B carrier status is associated with an increased risk of hepatocellular carcinoma

ANSWERS TO CASE 2.15

    iii. If mother is +ve for HBe antigen, the baby must receive hep B vaccination and immunoglobulin at birth

    v. HBe antibody positivity confers protection against transmission to baby

    x. Hepatitis B carrier status is associated with an increased risk of hepatocellular carcinoma

Carriers of HBsAg may have hepatitis B e antigen present (high infectivity, up to 90% mother-to-child transmission in some studies), or antibody to HBe (low infectivity, less than 5% perinatal transmission). Horizontal transmission between children also occurs.

If the mother has HBsAg and HBe antibody present, the baby should be given hepatitis B immunisation soon after birth and also at 1 and 6 months. If HbeAg is present (or HBe antibody is not present), the child should receive hepatitis B immunoglobulin within 24 h of birth, along with the immunisation schedule described. The immunoglobulin does not interfere with immunisation response.

Vertical transmission can be reduced by 90% by active immunisation at birth.

When hepatitis B is acquired as a neonate or infant, the risk of developing hepatitis B carrier status is very high. Carrier status is associated with an increased risk of hepatic cirrhosis and hepatocellular carcinoma in adult life, causing a million deaths annually worldwide. The WHO recommends that all countries immunise for hepatitis B as a part of their Expanded Program of Immunization (EPI), and currently, over 100 countries have implemented this. Hepatitis B immunisation is not currently a part of the routine immunisation schedule for children in the UK.

Any mother found to be positive for HbsAg should have her hepatitis B e antibody status checked, and if negative the HBe antigen status should be tested. The mother's liver function should be checked. She should be followed up, as we do not know how recently she acquired infection, and she may sero-convert. Antenatal screening should also include offering testing for syphilis and HIV.

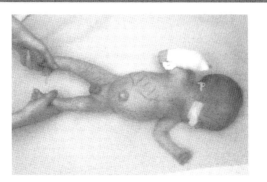

Fig 2.16

A 4-week-old boy presents to A&E with a small amount of bleeding from the umbilical stump. The child is exclusively breast fed and though generally well, is noted to be mildly jaundiced. He was born at term, birth weight 2800 g. The child is passing pale stools, and the child is shown in the photo. The clotting screen demonstrates a prothrombin time of 42 s (control 13), a partial thromboplastin time of 38 s (normal) and a normal fibrinogen count. The total bilirubin was 93 µmol/l with a conjugated bilirubin of 78 µmol/l.

The child's α-1antitrypsin level is 0.7 g/l (normal >1 g/l) and the phenotype is PIZZ.

What would you tell the parents regarding the child's prognosis?

SELECT *TWO* ANSWERS ONLY

   i. The prognosis is usually worse in females
  ii. The PIZZ phenotype is consistent with liver disease but rarely with pulmonary complications
 iii. There is a 50% chance that the baby will not have any long-term liver disease
 iv. There is a 1:4 chance of any subsequent children being affected
  v. There is a 50:50 chance of any subsequent male children being affected
 vi. Pulmonary manifestations occur before hepatic manifestations so he is unlikely to suffer any respiratory problems

ANSWERS TO CASE 2.16

a. iii. There is a 50% chance that the baby will not have any long-term liver disease
   iv. There is a 1:4 chance of any subsequent children being affected

When taking the history, it is important to ask about the antenatal history: any infections during pregnancy, consanguinity, and any family history of liver disease. One also needs to ask whether the child has had vitamin K. The most likely diagnoses would be biliary atresia or α-1 antitrypsin deficiency in view of the degree of cholestasis and the prolonged prothrombin time suggesting vitamin K deficiency. The intrauterine growth retardation in this context also suggests intrauterine infection or Alagille syndrome.

α-1 antitrypsin deficiency is the most common inherited cause of the neonatal hepatitis syndrome, occurring in 1:1600-2000 live births in European populations. Prenatal diagnosis by chorionic villous sampling is available. The children tend to have intrauterine growth retardation, often severe cholestasis and differentiation from biliary atresia can be difficult. Approximately 2% present with vitamin K responsive coagulopathy. The major manifestation of AAT deficiency in the first 2 decades of life is liver disease; pulmonary manifestations appear later. The PIZZ phenotype is responsible for nearly all cases of AAT emphysema and liver disease.

Initial emergency therapy should be initiated with the child being given parenteral vitamin K daily until the PT normalizes. If more severe bleeding develops, his coagulopathy should be corrected immediately with fresh frozen plasma. Thereafter management is supportive with nutritional intervention if failure to thrive occurs. Supplements of fat-soluble vitamins are required and follow-up, usually on a shared care basis with a paediatric gastroenterologist/liver centre, to monitor growth, disease progression and to ensure that further vitamin deficiencies do not occur.

Inheritance of α-1 antitrypsin deficiency is autosomal recessive. There is a 1:4 chance of any future child being affected and there is a poorer prognosis in males. The prognosis in α-1 antitrypsin deficiency is variable. Of those that present with early liver disease, approximately 50% do well with no progression to long-term liver disease, though some have a persisting transaminitis. In 25%, the liver disease progresses quickly and they require transplantation in the first year of life. In the other 25%, the liver disease progresses more slowly to cirrhosis and eventual decompensation requiring transplantation.

CASE 2.17

A 12-day-old girl is admitted to hospital with a short history of poor feeding, lethargy and jitteriness. She was born at term by normal vaginal delivery, with a birth weight of 3.5 kg and good Apgar scores. There were no risk factors for sepsis. The first day check was unremarkable, and she was discharged home on day 2. Two days prior to this admission, she was prescribed nasal drops by her GP for a snuffly nose. On examination she is pyrexial, tachycardic with a pulse of 150 bpm, normotensive, and has an oxygen saturation of 88% in air. Capillary refill time is 4 s. Cardiovascular examination is otherwise normal. Her respiratory rate is 60/min, although air entry is bilaterally good with minimal recession. Her abdomen is non-tender, with a 2 cm hepatomegaly and a normal umbilicus. ENT examination is unremarkable. She has a left exudative conjunctivitis but no rash. A self-limiting apnoea lasting 10 s was observed during the examination. The initial investigations revealed the following:

Hb 17.5 g/dl
WCC 5.1×10^9/l (neutrophils 2.3, lymphocytes 2.2)
Platelets 73×10^9/l
CRP 17 g/l
Glucose, electrolytes and renal function were normal
CXR and urinalysis are unremarkable
CSF negative Gram stain

Blood is taken for culture. The baby is commenced on oxygen, i.v. fluids, cefotaxime and gentamicin, and is observed on the high-dependency unit. On reassessment 6 h after admission, the infant is still tachycardic with a pulse of 160 bpm and now requires 50% headbox oxygen. She has a 6 cm hepatomegaly. Further investigations are as follows: AST 7305 IU/l, alkaline phosphatase 207 IU/l, total bilirubin 25 μmol/l, PT >200 s, APTT >200 s.

What is the most likely diagnosis on reassessment?

SELECT *ONE* ANSWER ONLY

  i. Tuberculous meningitis
 ii. Meningococcal meningitis
iii. Congenital heart disease
 iv. Intracranial haemorrhage
  v. Herpes simplex encephalitis
 vi. Inborn error of metabolism
vii. α1-antitrypsin deficiency

ANSWERS TO CASE 2.17

v. Herpes simplex encephalitis

On initial assessment, differential diagnosis must include bacterial sepsis (most likely Group B streptococcal sepsis), HSV infection, intracranial haemorrhage and respiratory syncytial virus (RSV) infection. When there is no rapid improvement, further investigations at this stage should include blood gases, LFTs, coagulation screen, cranial ultrasound, eye swabs for microscopy, culture and sensitivity and for viral immunofluorescence and a nasopharyngeal aspirate to exclude RSV.

The most likely diagnosis on reassessment is disseminated HSV infection, which causes hepatic involvement and thus deranged LFTs and coagulation screen.

Treatment is with high-dose intravenous acyclovir for 14–21 days. This child also needs immediate aggressive management of the coagulopathy and intensive care management of multi-organ failure. In this case, HSV type 2 was isolated from the eye swab and CSF.

Up to 80% of women with genital herpes have no lesions at the time of delivery and no known history of genital herpes and are not identified to receive preventive obstetric management or expectant paediatric input. Although the individual risk of HSV transmission in this group is very small, more than 70% of cases of neonatal HSV arise from this population of mothers. It follows, therefore, that, although a history of HSV in the mother is certainly helpful, its absence does not eliminate the risk of vertical transmission. Cutaneous manifestations of neonatal HSV infection (skin, eyes and mouth) require immediate intravenous acyclovir as there is a 70% risk of disseminated HSV infection or encephalitis without treatment. Disseminated neonatal HSV infection usually occurs in the first 14 days of life and typically presents with non-specific signs such as poor feeding, lethargy and fever. There are no cutaneous manifestations in 50% of cases. Dramatically elevated LFT results and a coagulopathy are common. The mortality is 74% with treatment. Disseminated neonatal HSV infection and antiviral treatment should be considered in all potentially septic neonates presenting during this period.

Questions and Answers for the New Format Exam

CASE 2.18

A 9-year-old girl is referred to the outpatient clinic with a 1-month history of weakness, lethargy, weight loss and sore legs. She has had great difficulty climbing the stairs over the past week, and her parents have resorted to carrying her. She is being bullied at school, and her parents think some of her symptoms may be psychosomatic. Further symptomatic enquiry is unremarkable. On examination she has periorbital violaceous erythema. She has a hoarse voice, is unable to lift her head off the pillow and has difficulty sitting upright. Cardiovascular, respiratory and abdominal system examination is unremarkable. The upper parts of her arms and legs are tender on palpation. Arm abduction and elbow flexion are grade 3/5 bilaterally. Other arm movements are normal. Hip flexion is grade 3/5 bilaterally, with otherwise normal leg movements. The knee jerk is reduced bilaterally; the ankle jerks are both normal and the plantar reflexes flexor. She is not ataxic.

Initial investigations revealed the following:
Hb 9.8 g/dl
WCC $4.4 \times 10^9/l$
Platelets $459 \times 10^9/l$
ESR 42 mm/hour
Na 138 mmol/l
K 4.2 mmol/l
Urea 2.9 mmol/l
Creatinine 55 µmol/l

What is the most likely diagnosis?

SELECT *ONE* ANSWER ONLY
  i. Guillain–Barre syndrome
 ii. Lyme disease
iii. Polymyalgia rheumatica
 iv. Systemic lupus erythematosus
  v. Dermatomyositis
 vi. Still's disease

ANSWERS TO CASE 2.18

v. Dermatomyositis

Dermatomyositis is a systemic vasculopathy characterised by focal myositis and cutaneous findings such as periorbital violaceous erythema and papules over the extensor surfaces, including the classical Gottron's papules over the dorsum of the hand. Skin involvement may precede myositis, and the onset of proximal muscle weakness may be insidious and difficult to recognise, and may eventually manifest as difficulty in standing or combing the hair. Upper airway muscle involvement may cause hoarseness, choking and aspiration. Impaired gastrointestinal smooth muscle may precipitate constipation, abdominal pain, diarrhoea and infarction. Cardiac conduction defects, dilated cardiomyopathy, hepatosplenomegaly, ocular involvement and seizures have also been reported. Calcinosis is not uncommon at presentation.

At diagnosis creatine kinase (CK), AST and lactate dehydrogenase are all elevated, and antinuclear antibody is positive (speckled pattern) in 60%. The ESR may be normal or elevated, with a normocytic anaemia and lymphopenia commonplace. ESR and CK value can be used to monitor the response to treatment. A paediatric rheumatologist should supervise management. The diagnostic yield of electromyography and muscle biopsy can be increased with the use of MRI to localise active disease, although these investigations are not needed when the diagnosis is clinically obvious, as in this case. Steroids are the mainstay of treatment. Pulsed methylprednisolone is reserved for those with severe disease (respiratory and palatal involvement) at presentation. Methotrexate and cyclophosphamide are alternatives in cases unresponsive to steroid therapy. Dysphagia may necessitate tubefeeding, and in rare cases of respiratory failure, tracheostomy and ventilation may be required. Physiotherapy and sunscreen are essential. With aggressive immunosuppressive therapy, the period of active symptoms is typically 18 months. The mortality is 3%, with long-term morbidity still under evaluation.

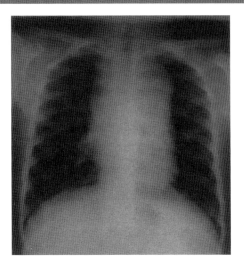

Fig 2.19

A 12-year-old boy is referred to A&E by his GP with a diagnosis of difficult asthma and acutely worsening shortness of breath. He was relatively well until about 6 weeks ago when he developed a dry cough and difficulty breathing, especially after exercise. There is a family history of atopy. The family has two cats, and both parents smoke. Despite being prescribed a salbutamol inhaler 6 weeks ago, he has also required two courses of oral prednisolone for his respiratory symptoms, these being of benefit on both occasions. He was started on becotide 200 mg two puffs twice daily 3 weeks ago. Because of occasional fever, his GP prescribed a 3 day course of azithromycin 2 weeks ago. Despite antibiotic treatment, his symptoms have progressed, and his mother says that his breathing at night is becoming noisier and noisier. He has been sleeping sitting up in bed for the past 5 days. On examination, he is afebrile with a pulse of 95 bpm and a respiratory rate of 40 per minute. His oxygen saturation in air is 93%. His chest is mildly hyperexpanded, and breath sounds are reduced bilaterally. There is a quiet biphasic stridor and intermittent expiratory wheeze. Cardiovascular examination is unremarkable. He has small mobile anterior cervical lymphadenopathy, an injected oropharynx and a spleen palpable to 3 cm below the costal margin. His CXR is shown.

What is the most likely diagnosis?

SELECT *ONE* ANSWER ONLY
  i. Hypertrophic obstructive cardiomyopathy
 ii. Haemomediastinum
iii. T-cell lymphoblastic lymphoma
 iv. Thoracic aortic aneurysm
  v. Pulmonary embolism
 vi. Bronchiectasis

ANSWERS TO CASE 2.19

iii. T-cell lymphoblastic lymphoma

The CXR shows a mediastinal mass, most likely to be a T-cell lymphoblastic lymphoma. Investigations should include a blood film, tissue diagnosis (lymph node biopsy and pleural aspirate), a bone marrow biopsy and a lumbar puncture.

The presentation of non-Hodgkin's lymphoma (NHL) depends primarily on the site of disease. T-cell lymphoblastic lymphoma most commonly (50-70%) presents with an anterior mediastinal mass. Local complications include compression of the intrathoracic airway giving rise to respiratory compromise and biphasic stridor, and compression of the superior vena cava causing SVC syndrome and pleural effusion. Rapid growth and early dissemination are typical of NHL so diagnosis, staging and initiation of treatment must be prompt. Tissue diagnosis must be made and can sometimes be difficult if the tumour is causing respiratory compromise as a general anaesthetic may be impossible. Diagnostic material can be obtained from pleural fluid, peripheral lymphadenopathy, bone marrow or CSF. T-cell NHL and T-cell ALL represent a spectrum of disease. By definition, if there is greater than 25% bone marrow infiltration the diagnosis is T-cell ALL. T-cell lymphoblastic lymphoma is exquisitely sensitive to steroid therapy, which will rapidly shrink a mediastinal mass. Tumour lysis syndrome is a common consequence of treatment and with large mediastinal tumours may even occur pretreatment if the tumour mass outgrows its blood supply. Pre-treatment creatinine, uric acid and lactate dehydrogenase (a marker of rapid cell turnover) need to be measured and the size of mediastinal mass assessed on imaging. Pre-treatment intravenous hydration and allopurinol are used to reduce the risk of tumour lysis syndrome.

A 2-week-old male infant was referred by his GP with a history of persistent vomiting, poor feeding, irritability and weight loss. His parents had also noted that he had been becoming increasingly drowsy over the previous few days. Examination revealed a mottled infant with a capillary refill time of 4 s. He was hypotonic and difficult to rouse, but apart from this, systemic examination was unremarkable. A full septic screen was performed, and the baby was commenced on broad-spectrum antibiotics. Blood, urine and CSF cultures were all negative. In view of this and the initial presenting picture, the possibility of a metabolic disorder was raised.

Further investigations were undertaken.

Which of the following results would suggest a diagnosis of an inborn error of metabolism?

SELECT *THREE* ANSWERS ONLY

   i. pCO_2 of 6 kPa
  ii. Serum Ca of 1.8 mmol/l
 iii. Serum bicarbonate of 14 mmol/l
 iv. Ammonia 40 µmol/l
  v. Lactate 0.8 mmol/l
 vi. pH of 7.34
 vii. Base excess −4 mmol/l
viii. Serum bicarbonate of 38 mmol/l
 ix. pH of 7.17
  x. Blood glucose of 1.8 mmol/l

ANSWERS TO CASE 2.20

iii. Serum bicarbonate of 14 mmol/l
ix. pH of 7.17
x. Blood glucose of 1.8 mmol/l

Factors in the history which would suggest an inborn error of metabolism (IEM) include poor feeding, irritability, persistent vomiting and drowsiness. Findings of metabolic acidosis and hypoglycaemia, and possibly deranged LFTs (raised transaminases) would also support this diagnosis.

Management consists of the following:

(1) Supportive care: intensive care if necessary; adequate respiratory support; the correction of hypothermia, hypoglycaemia and dehydration; monitoring electrolytes and blood gases; the correction of any metabolic acidosis with intravenous sodium bicarbonate (0.5-2 mmol/kg/hr); intravenous antibiotics as septicaemia is commonly associated with metabolic decompensation.

(2) Stopping all exogenous protein and giving intravenous glucose at 5-10 mg/kg/min in addition to insulin to promote anabolism and prevent catabolism.

(3) Further treatment depends upon the diagnosis.

Although inborn errors of metabolism are a significant cause of mortality and morbidity in children, with early recognition and appropriate treatment, the outcome can be good for many disorders. Making the correct diagnosis is also important in order to refer the family for genetic counselling; prenatal diagnosis is offered for subsequent pregnancies. An IEM should be suspected in a child of any age with any of the following: unexplained acute encephalopathy; progressive neurological disease; acid–base disturbance or hypoglycaemia; lactic acidaemia; certain dysmorphic features (e.g. Zellweger syndrome); unexplained multi-organ or single-organ disease.

Metabolic investigations are divided into three stages. First-line investigations are those which would normally be undertaken in any sick child but whose results may point towards the diagnosis of an IEM – blood gas, sugar, electrolytes (increased anion gap), LFTs and a full septic screen. Second-line investigations should be undertaken if an inborn error of metabolism is suspected and should be considered early in the course of the disease.

Table 2.20.1

Second-line investigations	Indications	Comment
Blood ammonia	Encephalopathy	Normal <80 μmol/l
Blood lactate	Encephalopathy, acidosis	Normal <2.5 mmol/l
Insulin, C-peptide, growth hormone cortisol	Hypoglycaemia	Endogenous hyperinsulinism
Urinary reducing substances	Liver/renal disease	Unreliable for diagnosis of galactosaemia
Urinary ketones	Encephalopathy, metabolic acidosis, hypoglycaemia	Marked ketosis is unusual in newborn and suggests an IEM
Acyl carnitines	Encephalopathy, metabolic acidosis, hypoglycaemia, hyperammonaemia	Fat oxidation defects, organic acidaemias
Urinary/plasma amino acids	Encephalopathy, hypoglycaemia, high ammonia level	Aminoacidopathies, urea cycle defects
Urinary organic acids	Encephalopathy, hypoglycaemia, hyperammonaemia	Fat oxidation defects, organic acidaemias
Plasma carnitine	Metabolic acidosis, hypoglycaemia, cardiomyopathy, encephalopathy84	Primary and secondary carnitine deficiencies
Beutler test	Liver disease	Screening for galactosaemia

Chapter

CASE 3.1

A 4-year-old girl presented with 'excessive thirst'. She was drinking 3 l during the day and waking at night asking for drinks. She was passing plenty of urine, but was not enuretic. She is otherwise well and has a 2-month-old brother.

Investigations:
Na 134 mmol/l
K 4.1 mmol/l
Ca 2.2 mmol/l

A water deprivation test showed the following:
Serum osmolality 292 mosmol/l
Urine osmolality 930 mosmol/l

a. What further investigations/results are initially necessary?
SELECT *TWO* ANSWERS ONLY
  i. CT head
  ii. Serum glucose
  iii. Glucose tolerance test
  iv. Serum urea and creatinine
  v. Renal ultrasound scan
  vi. Urine microscopy and culture

b. What is the most likely diagnosis?
SELECT *ONE* ANSWER ONLY
  i. Diabetes mellitus
  ii. Excessive salt intake
  iii. Nephrogenic diabetes insipidus
  iv. Cranial diabetes insipidus
  v. Psychogenic polydipsia

ANSWERS TO CASE 3.1

a. ii. Serum glucose
    iv. Serum urea and creatinine
b. v. Psychogenic polydipsia

Diabetes mellitus is a possible diagnosis as it often presents with polyuria and polydipsia. On examination, the child is not dehydrated and ketotic. It is excluded in this case by measuring serum glucose.

Chronic renal failure can present as polyuria (the kidneys are unable to concentrate the urine, producing urine of low osmolality) and consequent polydipsia. Features in the history may be suggestive such as recurrent urinary tract infections, but may well be absent.

Diabetes insipidus (DI) is excluded as she is able to concentrate her urine during the water deprivation test. This test must be undertaken with care, as a patient with true DI can rapidly become dehydrated.

Psychogenic polydipsia is common and the most likely diagnosis. It may be the symptom of emotional disturbance, in this case, the arrival of a new baby in the family.

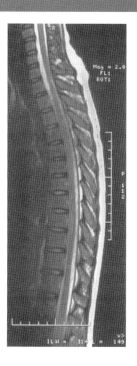

Fig 3.2

A 12-year-old girl developed rapidly progressive, lower limb weakness over 2 days. She initially noticed mild difficulties with walking and passing urine, despite the urge to void and was then rendered unable to walk. On examination, there was swelling of the optic discs, normal visual fields and otherwise no cranial nerve deficit. Power, tone, deep tendon reflexes and sensation were normal in the upper limbs. In the lower limbs, there were some anti-gravity movements in the hip flexors and adductors, but otherwise flaccid paresis distally and bilaterally in all other muscle groups. Knee and ankle jerks were exaggerated with ankle clonus and extensor plantar responses. Sensation was altered below a clear level at T5, with reduced perception of light touch and pinprick but preservation of vibration and position sense. Her bladder was palpable to the umbilicus; she was voiding small volumes of urine and therefore required catheterisation. Three weeks previously, she had an illness comprising sore throat and cervical lymphadenopathy. When questioned specifically, she could recall recently having an insect bite on her leg. She had previously been healthy. Her maternal grandmother had MS, diagnosed at age 18 years.

A lumbar puncture was performed after initial investigations. The results were as follows:

    CSF opening pressure 16 cm H_2O
    CSF protein 0.3 g/l
    CSF glucose 3.3 mmol/l
    CSF microscopy 16 white blood cells/high power field – 100% monocytes
    33 red blood cells/HPF
    Her MRI spine is shown

What is the most likely diagnosis?

SELECT *ONE* ANSWER ONLY

  i. Cerebral abscess
 ii. Acute transverse myelitis
iii. Spinal space-occupying lesion
 iv. Guillain–Barre syndrome
  v. Polyneuritis
 vi. Meningococcal disease

ANSWER TO CASE 3.2

ii. Acute transverse myelitis (ATM)

Differential diagnoses include a spinal space-occupying lesion (secondary to tumour, vascular malformation, abscess, haemorrhage or disease of the bony spine), or a vascular infarction of the cord (secondary to nucleus pulposus embolism or the primary anti-phospholipid syndrome). It is important initially to exclude spinal cord compression which may require urgent surgery.

Investigations include:
- brain and spinal cord imaging (to exclude spinal cord compression and raised intra-cranial pressure [before considering lumbar puncture])
- lumbar puncture (in ATM, usually lymphocyte pleocytosis, variably elevated protein, rarely more than three oligoclonal bands, normal glucose and pressure or CSF may be normal; in Guillain–Barre syndrome, pleocytosis is unlikely)
- PCR, CSF bacterial and viral culture, and intrathecal specific antibody serum serol-ogy throat swab, cultures of blood and stool
- ANF, rheumatoid factor, partial thromboplastin time, anticardiolipin antibody and antiphospholipid antibody
- B12 and prothrombin screen
- electrophysiology (may distinguish peripheral from CNS lesion but can be confusing early on if there is anterior horn cell involvement in ATM)

The MRI scan shows mild swelling or enlargement of the cord on T1 weighted images over T2-9, and ill-defined and patchy increased signal in the cord.

ATM is a condition of cord inflammation which can follow various triggers:
- post- or para-infectious inflammation (e.g. adenovirus, respiratory syncitial virus, influenza, measles, mumps and various vaccines)
- true invasion of the cord – rare, but suspect if there are matching general symptoms (e.g. varicella zoster, herpes simplex 1 and 2, Epstein–Barr virus, CMV, HIV, various coxsackie viruses, hepatitis A, borrelia vincenti, mycoplasma pneumoniae, yersinia enterocolitica, mycobacteria and parasites)
- systemic lupus erythematosus/other connective tissue diseases; thrombosis due to the anticardiolipin antibody
- lyme disease

The usual initial presentation in ATM is of sensory symptoms and bladder dysfunction with full-blown symptoms by 4 weeks. Severe back pain may occur at the beginning. There is usually a definite sensory level (80% thoracic). Sensory loss is often dissociated (loss of pain, temperature and light touch but preservation of position sense and vibra-tion). The degree of paraparesis varies considerably. Anterior horn cells may be involved and reflexes may be reduced or absent, later brisk. GBS may be a differential diagnosis when there is anterior horn cell involvement – tetraparesis and respiratory muscle involvement is more common, the sensory level usually less clear and early sphincter involvement unusual.

Treatment: high-dose i.v. steroid pulse therapy over 3 days is promising but unproven (dose regimen 20 mg/kg/day prednisolone or methylprednisolone). A pilot study has suggested earlier and more complete recovery with this regime. Rehabilitation should be established early on. Urodynamics and nephrology expertise may be required in cases of neuropathic bladder.

A 34 year-old known i.v. drug-abusing pregnant woman is found to be hepatitis C antibody and PCR positive. She is negative for HIV and hepatitis B. She asks to speak to you as the paediatrician for advice on the risks to the baby.

What advice should you give the mother?

SELECT *THREE* ANSWERS ONLY

i. There is no evidence that breast feeding increases the risk of chronic hepatitis C infection in the child
ii. Fetal scalp blood monitoring should be avoided during labour
iii. Evidence suggests that the baby should be delivered by Caesarean section
iv. A positive hepatitis C antibody at 1 year of age is diagnostic of infection with hepatitis C
v. There is a 20% risk of the child being chronically infected with hepatitis C
vi. Tests for hepatitis C can be carried out on the baby at birth (PCR)
vii. Hepatitis C virus is present in breast milk
viii. Hepatitis C antibody test at 6 months of age is diagnostic of infection

ANSWERS TO CASE 3.3

    i. There is no evidence that breast feeding increases the risk of chronic hepatitis infection in the child

    ii. Fetal scalp blood monitoring should be avoided during labour

    vii. Hepatitis C virus is present in breast milk

The risk of the child being chronically infected with hepatitis C is approximately 5%.

Presently, there is no compelling evidence suggesting that hepatitis C positive mothers should have elective Caesarean sections to reduce the infection risk to the child, but it is probably advisable to avoid fetal scalp blood monitoring during labour.

Despite a theoretical risk of infection from breast feeding (hepatitis C virus is present in breast milk), there is no evidence that breast feeding increases the risk of chronic hepatitis C infection in the child. This must be tempered, however, with the fact that the studies have been relatively small and a small increase in risk would not have been detected.

Possible tests are hepatitis C antibody and hepatitis C PCR on the child; hepatitis C antibody at 18 months or hepatitis C antibody and PCR at 6 months (to be repeated at 1 year if either is positive).

The prevalence of hepatitis C infection is as high as 80% in some drug-abusing populations. All present/past i.v. drug-abusing pregnant mothers should be screened for hepatitis C. The ideal testing policy for infants of hepatitis C positive mothers is difficult as children who do not develop chronic hepatitis C can have hepatitis C antibody for up to 16 months. Therefore, if one is to test for hepatitis C antibody alone, the test should be deferred until the child is 18 months old. The hepatitis C PCR test has a low sensitivity in the first month of life, but its sensitivity increases to approximately 97% from 1 month. Thus, a combination of hepatitis C antibody and PCR could be performed at 6 months with the proviso that if either were positive, then they would have to be repeated later. The prognosis of chronic hepatitis C in children is unknown, but hepatitis C is now the most common indication for adult liver transplantation. There are presently paediatric trials of combination therapy in chronic hepatitis C with interferon a and ribavirin. Although the treatment is unpleasant, the sustained viral clearance rates are likely to be similar to that in adults of ~50%.

CASE 3.4

A 21-day-old male infant of consanguineous parents was referred by his GP with collapse, vomiting and dehydration. He had no relevant antenatal history, and had been born normally at term and breast fed. There were no dysmorphic features, and he was estimated to be 10-15% dehydrated clinically. The infant was apyrexial, and there was no rash. His capillary refill time was 8 s.

Initial tests reveal the following:
Na 116 mmol/l
K 7.9 mmol/l
Urea 18 mmol/l
Chloride 85 mmol/l
pH 7.08
pCO_2 4.7 kPa
Base excess −15 mmol/l
Glucose 1.2 mmol/l

What are the key diagnostic tests of choice to be performed now?

SELECT *TWO* ANSWERS ONLY
 i. Abdominal ultrasound scan
 ii. Serum cortisol
 iii. U&E
 iv. Blood gas
 v. Serum 17-hydroxyprogesterone
 vi. Testosterone
 vii. Urinary steroid profile
 viii. Blood glucose
 ix. Karyotype

ANSWERS TO CASE 3.4

v. Serum 17-hydroxyprogesterone
vii. Urinary steroid profile

The most likely diagnosis here is a salt–losing crisis caused by congenital adrenal hyper-plasia (CAH). The three cardinal features of this potentially fatal condition are hyponat-raemia, hyperkalaemia and hypovolaemia, and this infant requires prompt resuscitation. Acute vomiting resulting from sepsis is less likely.

CAH is a group of disorders. The most common is the defect caused by 21-hydroxylase deficiency (between 1/5000 and 15000 births); it is more common in certain ethnic groups (Ashkenazi Jews). Other defects causing CAH (e.g. 11β-hydroxylase deficiency) are 10 times less frequent. 21-hydroxylase deficiency predisposes to crises as it affects both cortisol and aldosterone production. A lowered cortisol level stimulates ACTH production and consequent adrenal hyperplasia, the production of excessive androgens from the adrenals causing virilization of females; boys usually appear normal.

The key diagnostic tests are serum 17-hydroxyprogesterone (17-OHP) and urinary metabolites of 17-OHP. (You throw away marks if you repeat urea and electrolyte tests, gas levels and glucose readings as you have already done them!) It will be neces-sary to check that the child is male (and not a virilized female) by ultrasound of the genitalia and by karyotyping. Inheritance is autosomal recessive; careful family history should be sought and parental counselling given. Further tests for mutations in the 21-hydroxylase gene can be performed.

This infant presented with hypovolaemic shock and initial management involved sta-bilising ABC; gaining i.v. access, and giving 20 ml/kg normal saline followed by a glucose bolus and infusion. Broad-spectrum i.v. antibiotics must be given, and intra-venous hydrocortisone is life-saving. Essential further investigations include a FBC and film, C-reactive peptide, blood and urine (SPA) cultures, and group and save. Urinary electrolytes will be helpful in this case (a high sodium level will be noted).

Treatment cornerstones include the following:
- Glucocorticoid replacement – hydrocortisone is the usual choice in children, reduc-ing androgen production by inhibition of ACTH and corticotrophin releasing hormone. It has less effect on growth than do other steroids such as prednisolone because of its short half-life.
- Mineralocorticoid replacement – if there is salt wasting, salt supplements (about 6-8 mmol/kg/day) and fludrocortisone are the usual treatment regimen.
- Surgery is occasionally used for genital anomalies; the usual aim is to raise affected children as their genetic sex, and in a few females clitoroplasty may be necessary.
- Other – it is important to mention that these children and their parents will require psychological counselling.
- Follow-up – these children should preferably be referred to a paediatric endocrinol-ogy service as they will require life-long follow-up.

CASE 3.5

A 10-year-old prepubertal boy was diagnosed with a medullablastoma. He was treated with surgery, chemotherapy and craniospinal radiotherapy (total cranial radiation dose: 5500 cGy). He was investigated for poor growth 2 years post-treatment with a glucagon stimulation test.

TSH 1.3 mU/l (normal range 0.5-6.0 mU/l)

Thyroxine 67 nmol/l (normal range 70-180 nmol/l)

Comment on the results of the stimulation test (Table 3.5.1).

SELECT *TWO* ANSWERS ONLY

 i. GH response within normal range
 ii. A low peak GH response
 iii. Inadequate glucose response
 iv. No evidence of GH deficiency
 v. Test inconclusive because of poor glucose response
 vi. Adequate cortisol response (>double at 2 h)
 vii. Satisfactory glucose response

Table 3.5.1

Time (mins)	Glucose (mmol/l)	GH (mU/l)	Cortisol (nmol/l)
0	4.5	4.5	85
30	7.5	3.9	140
60	5.0	3.6	136
90	3.3	4.0	141
120	4.7	6.4	199
150	4.7	3.6	149
180	4.6	3.2	115

ANSWERS TO CASE 3.5

  ii. A low peak GH response
 vii. Satisfactory glucose response

The test produced a satisfactory glucose response to glucagon with an initial rise of blood glucose and a fall of >2 mmol/l. The peak GH response is low at 6.4 mU/l (normal range >20 mU/l) signifying GH insufficiency.

Doses of cranial radiation in excess of 3000 cGy are almost all associated with GH deficiency within 5 years. There is a more variable outcome with lower doses, with some patients having neurosecretory dysfunction. The cortisol levels do not satisfy the criteria for an adequate response, i.e. low baseline value (normal range >120-150 nmol/l), the cortisol level fails to rise 200 nmol/l above the baseline and the peak value does not exceed 500 nmol/l. This boy is at risk of both primary and secondary hypothyroidism. Damage to the thyroid gland may result from scatter radiation following spinal radiotherapy, which leads to primary hypothyroidism (raised TSH, low/normal thyroxine). Damage to the hypothalamic-pituitary tract from cranial radiation can lead to secondary hypothyroidism (low TSH, low thyroxine). This patient received GH, hydrocortisone and thyroxine replacement.

Causes of abnormal linear growth include GH deficiency, hypothyroidism and hypocortisolaemia. He is also at risk of a subnormal pubertal growth spurt and a reduction in sitting height due to spinal radiation.

CASE 3.6

A mother brings her baby to clinic for his 6-week check. This is her first baby and the infant is bottle feeding on cows' milk formula. The mother is very anxious stating that the baby cries constantly, does not feed and is not gaining weight. She thinks his milk should be changed. On further questioning, you find that the infant was born at 34 weeks' gestation (birth weight 2.1 kg, 25th centile) and spent 6 days on the special care baby unit where there were no complications apart from jaundice requiring 24 h phototherapy and nasogastric feeds for the first 2 days of life. The mother initially attempted to breast feed but stopped after 2 weeks as she felt she did not have enough milk. On examination, you find a well-looking, alert baby whose height, weight and head circumference all lie on the 25th centile.

a. What investigation must be done in this case?
    SELECT *ONE* ANSWER ONLY
  i. FBC and U&E
 ii. Thyroid function tests
iii. Stool for reducing substances
 iv. pH study
  v. Urine for microscopy and culture
 vi. None

b. What is the most likely diagnosis?
    SELECT *ONE* ANSWER ONLY
  i. Lactose intolerance
 ii. Gastro-oesophageal reflux
iii. Normal baby
 iv. Coeliac disease
  v. Cows' milk protein intolerance

ANSWERS TO CASE 3.6

a. vi. None
b. iii. Normal baby

In analysing feeding problems, it is important to enquire about the food, the delivery system and the recipient.

Food:

What type? (first or follow-on milk — advice may be required); how much? (overfeeding is a common problem); how often? (a frequent response to crying is to offer milk).

Delivery system:

Bottles may be difficult to clean — requires advice and suitable facilities; teats — need to adapt to suit the individual baby; are feeds being made up correctly?

Recipient:

Babies vary — some gobble and some are difficult feeders; the definition of infantile colic is an otherwise well baby with inconsolable crying for over 3 h a day.

It is also important to enquire about the mother's health and well-being. For instance, has she sufficient support and help with caring for the demands of a newborn infant, or has she symptoms of depression or other medical problems following the birth? Also ask if there are any other features in the infant, such as vomiting, loose stools or constipation, skin rashes or any significant family history. The causes of feeding problems which may be considered are as follows:

Concern the milk does not suit — Certain features may suggest cows' milk hypersensitivity. These include perioral swelling every time milk enters the mouth, retching and vomiting after a feed and colic associated with loose, sometimes blood-streaked stool. If this is suspected, soya feeds may be substituted but sensitivity to soya protein also occurs. Lactose sensitivity may present with diarrhoea which continues after gastroenteritis.

Regurgitation and vomiting — It is important to note the timing of reflux in relation to feeding, the volume lost, whether the infant seems uncomfortable and whether they are thriving.

Anxiety that the infant is not getting enough — This is common and often leads to overfeeding, vomiting and further anxiety. Reassurance plus a careful analysis of the growth chart to demonstrate normal weight gain to the parents is helpful.

If, after careful questioning and examination, there are no features to suggest any disease in the infant, the correct management is maternal reassurance, addressing and allaying her worries, together with support from the health visitor.

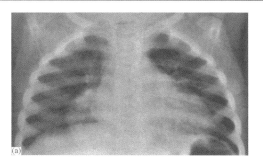

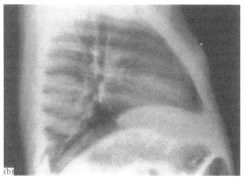

Fig 3.7

A 3-year-old girl attended with a 2-day history of sore throat, lethargy, anorexia, cough and occasional vomiting but no diarrhoea. Initial vital signs were: temperature 39.6°C, SaO$_2$ 96% in room air, respiratory rate 35/min, pulse 140 bpm. She was lethargic but interacted well. Her pharynx was injected. Chest examination showed symmetrical air entry with no added sounds. The abdomen was soft, but with diffuse non-localised tenderness. Neurological examination was normal. FBC showed a normal haemoglobin and platelet count. WBC was 18 × 10^9/l with a predominant neutrophilia. A CXR was performed.

What abnormality does the CXR show?

SELECT THE MOST LIKELY ANSWER

  i. Cardiomegaly
  ii. Round pneumonia
  iii. Right atrial enlargement
  iv. Mediastinal mass
  v. Right middle lobe collapse

Questions and Answers for the New Format Exam

ANSWER TO CASE 3.7

ii. Round pneumonia

The CXR shows a well-defined, rounded, soft tissue opacity in the right lower zone which is a 'round pneumonia'. Round pneumonias are often caused by Streptococcus pneumoniae (pneumococcus). Most children with pneumonia can be managed as outpatients using oral therapy. For community acquired pneumonia where pneumococcal infection is suspected, amoxycillin is probably now the drug of choice. Indications for inpatient care include systemic toxicity, underlying immune deficiency, dehydration, the need for oxygen therapy (SaO_2 <93%), social vulnerability and poor clinical response to initial treatment. Round pneumonias are usually located in the posterior and lower lobes of the lung. Their appearance and location may raise concern about the possibility of an intrathoracic tumour, especially of neurogenic origin. Radiologically the edges of a round pneumonia are usually less well defined than those of a tumour, and an air bronchogram may be present. The typical clinical presentation and rapid response to antibiotic treatment such as benzylpenicillin or amoxycillin should make the diagnosis clear. Follow-up CXR, usually only justified in situations of initial lobar collapse, may give final reassurance.

CASE 3.8

A 5-year-old boy was referred to the community paediatric services by his teacher. Development in all areas was satisfactory until the boy started school. His teacher noted that his academic progress had slowed, and he began to exhibit behavioural and concentration difficulties. He also appeared to have hearing difficulties, and his speech became less comprehensible. At presentation, he had severe problems affecting receptive language, expressive language and speech sounds. His development in other areas appeared satisfactory. There were no concerns from his past medical or birth history.

General and neurological examinations – satisfactory

EEG/sleep EEG – frequent left-sided epileptiform discharges, much more frequent during sleep

Hearing assessment – normal

Cranial MRI – normal

What is the probable diagnosis?

SELECT *ONE* ANSWER ONLY

   i. Benign Rolandic epilepsy
  ii. West syndrome
 iii. Landau–Kleffner syndrome
 iv. Mitochondrial myopathy
  v. Lennox–Gastaut syndrome

ANSWER TO CASE 3.8

iii. Landau–Kleffner syndrome (LKS)

LKS, also known as acquired epileptic aphasia, is a rare form of childhood epilepsy resulting in a severe language disorder. It usually develops between 3 and 8 years of age. In most cases, development is normal up to this age. The rate of development of this syndrome is very variable. In young children who have not learned to talk, it may be mistaken for a developmental language disorder, deafness or autism. All children with LKS have abnormal electrical activity in one or both temporal areas, the areas of the brain responsible for processing language. Epileptiform activity is evident on EEG testing, particularly during sleep. Approximately two-thirds of children have night seizures.

The language disorder usually affects comprehension. Many children have difficulty in understanding their own name. They are also likely to have difficulty recognising environmental sounds such as a ringing telephone. These children may appear to be deaf. Expressive language can also be affected, and some children completely lose their speech. A child may rarely understand language but have difficulty speaking.

Behavioural problems especially hyperactivity, poor attention, depression and irritability, are common. Some have episodes of very abnormal 'autistic type behaviour'. The behaviour, seizures and the epileptiform EEG usually resolve by early adolescence. Some may fully recover their language, but many are left with a disability. Paediatric neurology referral is required. Referral should also be made to the speech and language therapist and educational psychologist.

Treatment options include steroids, antiepileptic drugs and neurosurgery.

Antiepileptic drugs are used to treat seizures but may not affect the EEG abnormalities in the long term. Steroids taken early or for a sufficient time often improve the EEG findings and allow language to recover. For those who do not respond to these measures, neurosurgery (multiple subpial transection) may be appropriate. Appropriate speech and language therapy and special education are essential.

An introduction to sign language may be required.

CASE 3.9

A 14-year-old boy arrived in hospital with status epilepticus. He had had surgical repair of a lumbosacral myelomeningocoele in infancy and had had a decompression of the foramen magnum for Arnold–Chiari malformation 2 months before this admission. The seizure was treated with intravenous diazepam and phenytoin. On examination, he was agitated with a Glasgow coma score of 9, pulse 70/min and his blood pressure was 200/120 mm hg. His electrolytes were as follows:

Na 137 mmol/l
K 4.1 mmol/l
Urea 21 mmol/l
Creatinine 364 µmol/l
Bicarbonate 17.5 mmol/l
Glucose 10.5 mmol/l

What is the likely cause of his raised blood pressure?

SELECT *ONE* ANSWER ONLY

  i. Hypertensive encephalopathy secondary to chronic renal failure
 ii. Raised intracranial pressure secondary to obstructive hydrocephalus
iii. Phenytoin ingestion
iv. Acute tubular necrosis secondary to poor renal perfusion in status epilepticus

ANSWERS TO CASE 3.9

i. Hypertensive encephalopathy secondary to chronic renal failure

This boy had hypertensive encephalopathy secondary to chronic renal failure. In his case, the most likely cause of renal failure is obstructive uropathy caused by a neuropathic bladder.

A CT head scan should be performed to look for signs of raised intracranial pressure or post-operative complications, e.g. bleeding. This will necessitate intubation and ventilation in view of his reduced conscious level and agitation.

A labetolol infusion is used to treat the hypertension by a controlled reduction, initially at a rate of 1–3 mg/kg/h. Invasive monitoring of blood pressure via an arterial line may be required. Other drugs used include hydralazine and nifedipine. This boy also requires catheterisation and is likely to need long-term intermittent self-catheterisation.

An 11-year-old boy was referred by the school nurse for investigation of his short stature. He was born on the 50th percentile for height but on presentation was below the 3rd percentile. As a baby, he suffered from gastro-oesophageal reflux, recurrent vomiting and failure to thrive. He walked at 20 months. He was thought to be clumsy and diagnosed as dyspraxic. General examination revealed a prominent chest, low posterior hairline and small-volume testes. His bone age was 8 years.

a. What is the probable diagnosis?
SELECT *ONE* ANSWER ONLY
 i. Angelman syndrome
 ii. Prader–Willi syndrome
 iii. Mitochondrial cytopathy
 iv. Beckwith–Wiedemann syndrome
 v. Noonan syndrome
 vi. William's syndrome

b. What other investigation is essential?
SELECT *ONE* ANSWER ONLY
 i. Abdominal ultrasound scan
 ii. Growth hormone
 iii. Electroencephalogram
 iv. Echocardiogram
 v. Serum Calcium

ANSWERS TO CASE 3.10

a. v. Noonan syndrome
b. iv. Echocardiogram

Noonan syndrome was first described in 1963. The overall incidence of the condition is between 1:1000 and 1:2500 live births. Although the inheritance is autosomal dominant, many cases are sporadic. A gene mutation of the PTPN11 (protein-tyrosine phosphatase, non-receptor-type 11) gene underlying this condition has been located on chromosome 12 and is found in about 50% of cases.

Noonan syndrome is a clinical diagnosis. It is characterised by dysmorphic facial features (hypertelorism, downwards-slanting palpebral fissures, ptosis, low-set and posteriorly rotated ears, a low posterior hairline and a short neck), short stature and cardiovascular anomalies (pulmonary valvular stenosis, hypertrophic cardiomyopathy and atrial septal defect). Chest deformity (pectus carinatum/excavatum), low-set nipples, cryptorchidism, mild motor delay and learning difficulty are also frequent associations. Bleeding diatheses (a prolonged APTT and various coagulation factor deficiencies), gut dysmotility, hearing and visual abnormalities can also occur. Developmental co-ordination disorder (previously known as dyspraxia) occurs in more than 50% of affected children.

GH treatment improves height velocity in the short term. Long-term treatment has not, however, substantially improved final height.

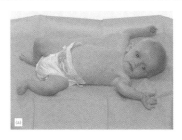
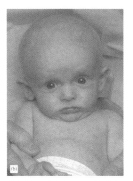

Fig 3.11

A 3-month-old male infant presented with failure to gain weight. There was no family history of note and the parents were not consanguineous. He was born full term and weighed 2700 g (9th centile). His head circumference and length were also on the 9th centile at birth. At 3 months, he weighed 4000 g, well below 0.4th centile, as were his head circumference and length. He was admitted to the ward for observation and assessment. He fed extremely well and took up to 200 ml/kg/day of bottle milk. On examination, he appeared dysmorphic. He was neither cyanosed nor icteric. He looked well and was not breathless at rest. He had a grade 2/6-ejection systolic murmur at the upper left sternal edge. His peripheral pulses were normal. He had a soft 2 cm liver edge palpable. His abdomen was not distended. He had normal tone and he was developing normally. Initial LFT showed:

ALP 1094 IU/l (100-300)
AST 100 IU/l (545)
Gamma GT 670 IU/l (10-120)
Bilirubin 8 μmol/l (1-22)
Total protein 74 g/l (55-75)
Albumin 45 g/l (35-50)

What is the likely syndrome?

SELECT *ONE* ANSWER ONLY

   i. Rubinstein–Taybi syndrome
  ii. Schwachmann syndrome
 iii. α1-antitrypsin deficiency
 iv. Alagille syndrome
  v. William's syndrome

ANSWERS TO CASE 3.11

iv. Alagille syndrome

This child is dysmorphic with deep-set eyes, a broad forehead, bulbous nose and prominent chin. He has poor growth and has an obstructive pattern to his LFTs. He has a cardiac murmur loudest in the pulmonary area. These features suggest Alagille syndrome (arteriohepatic dysplasia). Symptoms include an intrahepatic paucity of bile ducts with subsequent cholestasis, and a pulmonary artery stenosis, although patients can have atrial or ventricular septal defects or coarctation. Alagille syndrome patients have eye abnormalities including a posterior embryotoxon (prominence of Schwalbe's line). They may have reduced renal function with raised uric acid. If there were any doubt in his syndromic diagnosis, other causes of cholestatic liver disease would need to be explored.

Nutritional assessment is mandatory with particular focus on fat-soluble vitamins. Supplementation of these vitamins (A, D, E, K) is essential. Clotting studies should be checked. Hypercholesterolaemia is often associated with the syndrome. Review by a hepatology team is also required; ultrasound of the liver will confirm if there is an extrahepatic bile system and consideration for liver biopsy at some stage is required to demonstrate the biliary hypoplasia. Fluorescence in-situ hybridisation studies may demonstrate a deletion on chromosome 20p. The family will need genetic consultation. Ophthalmology assessment is required. Cardiac assessment in this case revealed a bilateral branch pulmonary artery stenosis, which was uncomplicated. Renal function needs to be monitored and some children may get further growth retardation secondary to reduced GH or hypothyroidism.

Pruritis due to increased serum bile acids can cause major discomfort to the child.

The management options are: ursodeoxycholic acid (10-20 mg/kg/day divided), phenobarbitone (3-5 mg/kg/day), rifampicin (3-10 mg/kg/day) or trimeprazine (dose dependent on age).

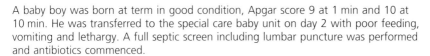

A baby boy was born at term in good condition, Apgar score 9 at 1 min and 10 at 10 min. He was transferred to the special care baby unit on day 2 with poor feeding, vomiting and lethargy. A full septic screen including lumbar puncture was performed and antibiotics commenced.

Over the next 12 h he deteriorated and required intubation for apnoeas. He subsequently had several right-sided seizures. He was noted to have 3 cm hepatomegaly and to be hypotonic. He was thoroughly investigated; results included ammonia 2500 μmol/l (normal 10-40) and raised serum and urine citrulline.

a. Which group of metabolic disorders does this condition belong to?
   SELECT *ONE* ANSWER ONLY
   i. Organic acidaemias
   ii. Mucopolysaccharidoses
   iii. Mitochondrial cytopathies
   iv. Mucolipidoses
   v. Urea cycle disorders
   vi. Glycogen storage diseases
   vii. Fatty acid oxidation defect

b. How could you manage his acute hyperammonaemia?
   SELECT *TWO* ANSWERS ONLY
   i. Forced alkaline diuresis
   ii. Stop intake of protein
   iii. Sodium phenylbutyrate
   iv. High protein diet
   v. TPN
   vi. Sodium bicarbonate

ANSWERS TO CASE 3.12

a. v. Urea cycle disorder
b. ii. Stop intake of protein
   iii. Sodium phenylbutyrate

This child has citrullinaemia, one of the urea cycle disorders. Abnormalities in the urea cycle create increased levels of ammonia, which cannot be metabolised. Urgent management is required to reduce these dangerous levels of ammonia. Measures include:

- Stop exogenous protein
- Inhibit catabolism of protein by giving maintenance glucose infusions, correcting any metabolic acidosis, reversing any hypothermia and treating seizures with anti-convulsant medication
- Use i.v. drugs to convert nitrogen to an excretable product: sodium benzoate, sodium phenylbutyrate and/or arginine can be used
- Dialysis (haemodialysis or peritoneal dialysis) is used if urine output is poor, ammonia levels are very high, or there is inadequate response to i.v. therapy

Long-term management involves the use of a low-protein diet, an emergency high-calorie regime during intercurrent illnesses to prevent protein catabolism and the use of oral medication to aid nitrogen excretion (e.g. arginine, sodium benzoate). Long-term prognosis, particularly in terms of mental handicap, is related to the avoidance of severe hyperammonaemia.

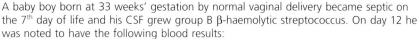

A baby boy born at 33 weeks' gestation by normal vaginal delivery became septic on the 7th day of life and his CSF grew group B β-haemolytic streptococcus. On day 12 he was noted to have the following blood results:

Na 165 mmol/l
K 4.5 mmol/l
Urea 6.8 mmol/l
Creatinine 52 μmol/l
Cortisol 28 nmol/l (on three consecutive samples)
TSH 3.54 miU/l
FT$_4$ 6.9 pmol/l

What is the most likely diagnosis?

SELECT *ONE* ANSWER ONLY

  i. Iatrogenic sodium overload
 ii. Acute tubular necrosis
iii. Bartter syndrome
 iv. Adrenal ischaemia
  v. Panhypopituitarism
 vi. Syndrome of inappropriate ADH secretion

ANSWERS TO CASE 3.13

i. Panhypopituitarism

This baby's blood results show hypernatraemia, with low cortisol and low thyroid hormone levels. This is consistent with a diagnosis of panhypopituitarism with diabetes insipidus. The cause of this is the group B strep meningitis.

Management involves replacement of deficient hormones – hydrocortisone and thyroxine (oral preparations) and desmopressin (synthetic analogue of arginine vasopressin which has a prolonged antidiuretic effect and almost absent pressor activity) for diabetes insipidus. The route of administration for desmopressin could be intranasal or oral. The oral preparation, however, is not as effective as the nasal preparation.

General advice should be given to the carers regarding intercurrent illness, stress or physical effort, which will increase the requirement of hydrocortisone. Training must be given to parents and registration with the local paramedics is required for administration of intramuscular hydrocortisone which is needed prior to reaching the hospital in cases where the child has a serious illness (e.g. fractured femur, sepsis, etc.). The foremost rule in the treatment of diabetes insipidus is that the child should have access to water or fluids. This is more important in infancy when the child is unable to ask for water. The family must be informed that during the replacement therapy the child is unprotected against excess water. If severe ill health occurs during combined hydrocortisone and ADH treatment then stop the DDAVP treatment during the period of steroid dose increase, and restrict fluid intake to avoid dilutional hyponatraemia – restart the DDAVP only when a diuresis occurs.

Education of the family is of prime importance. A Medic-alert bracelet with the diagnosis and treatment is strongly recommended.

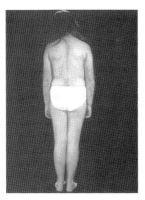

Fig 3.14.a

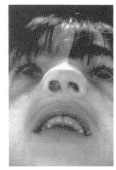

Fig 3.14.b

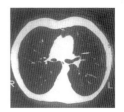

Fig 3.14.c

A 5-year-old girl with CF underwent a heart–lung transplant. At the regular review in the outpatient clinic, she presented with the features illustrated in Figure 3.14.a, b.

a. What is the aetiology of these features?
SELECT *ONE* ANSWER ONLY
  i. Vitamin A deficiency
  ii. CF related disease
  iii. Graft versus host disease
  iv. Immunosuppressant therapy

Three years after the transplant, she presented with history of progressive shortness of breath and a reduction in exercise tolerance, and this CT scan (Fig. 3.14.c) was performed.

b. What is the most likely diagnosis?
SELECT *ONE* ANSWER ONLY
  i. Obliterative bronchiolitis
  ii. Allergic bronchopulmonary aspergillosis
  iii. Pulmonary oedema
  iv. Pneumocystis carinii

ANSWERS TO CASE 3.14

a. iv. Immunosuppressant therapy
b. i. Obliterative bronchiolitis (OB)

The features illustrated are hirsutism, nasal polyps and gingival hypertrophy. All three are cyclosporin-related side-effects, although nasal polyps may also be found in CF. Management options include the practical measures of use of a depilatory cream, gum shaving and polypectomy, while maintaining the patient free from rejection on a minimal dose of cyclosporin. An alternative would be switching cyclosporin to tacrolimus (FK 506). Both have a similar mechanism of action (inhibiting T-cell synthesis of lymphokines, hence activation and proliferation of cell-mediated cytotoxicity and humoral immunity) but changes to physical appearance are not a side-effect of tacrolimus.

OB is the pathological hallmark of chronic graft dysfunction. The CT scan demonstrates bronchial dilatation, decreased peripheral vascular markings and a hyperinflated chest. These findings are most consistent with a diagnosis of OB. There are many processes (allo-immune and non allo-immune) which lead to fibrotic obliteration of airway lumen. The average time to onset or diagnosis is 16-20 months but the range can be very broad. The clinical presentation can be acute and imitate infection, or insidious with a progressive decline in lung function. The diagnosis of OB is complemented by transbronchial biopsy and spirometry. Recurrent acute rejection is the most significant risk factor. CMV infection or pneumonia is also believed to be a predisposing factor. But the precursor pathophysiology is not clear. Once OB has occurred, it is rarely fully arrested by therapy and the response is often transient.

Management consists of immunosuppressant therapy. In the UK, the most widely used triple immunosuppressant regimen is cyclosporin, azathioprine and prednisolone.

CASE 3.15

A baby weighing 1800 g was born by emergency Caesarean section for pregnancy-induced hypertension at 31 weeks' gestation. From day 4 of life, he became progressively jaundiced. He had mild respiratory distress syndrome, presumed necrotising enterocolitis that was being treated conservatively, and had received total parenteral nutrition. He was the first child of healthy parents, and the mother's blood group was O positive. His length and weight were below the 0.4th centile, and his head circumference on the 2nd centile. Examination revealed a splenic tip and a 1 cm smooth liver edge.

His blood tests on day 20 were as follows:
Haemoglobin 16.7 g/dl
Total bilirubin 151 μmol/l
Conjugated bilirubin 132 μmol/l
ALP 350 IU/l
ALT 58 IU/l
Albumin 28 g/l

There is one important diagnosis which initially needs excluding; what investigation would need to be carried out to exclude this?

SELECT *ONE* ANSWER ONLY
  i. Coagulation screen
  ii. Urobilinogen
  iii. Liver biopsy
  iv. Hepatogram
  v. Liver ultrasound scan
  vi. HIDA scan
  vii. Fungal blood cultures

ANSWER TO CASE 3.15

vi. HIDA scan

The differential diagnosis includes sepsis, biliary atresia, TPN-related hepatitis, and physiological jaundice. Prolonged i.v. nutrition causes cholestasis and hepatocellular damage, which may progress to cirrhosis. Prevalence increases with the degree of prematurity, degree of intra-uterine growth retardation and duration of parenteral nutrition. Sepsis, hypoxia, intraabdominal surgery and hepatotoxic drugs aggravate the damage.

Other important factors from the history are stool colour and urine colour. This is to help differentiate between obstructive and non-obstructive jaundice. In obstructive jaundice, the stools would be pale and the urine would be dark.

Biliary atresia is the condition which needs prompt diagnosis as if caught early enough it is amenable to treatment. This is a destructive sclerosing inflammatory process extending from the extrahepatic biliary tree to the intrahepatic ducts. Its incidence is approximately one in 14 000 live births. Prevalence is the same in premature and term babies. Surgical correction (Kasai operation) by 60 days of age is the gold-standard treatment. Surgery is usually postponed until the baby reaches 3000 g, as the risk of surgery is too great earlier. Either a Kasai operation may be carried out or a liver transplant performed. Investigations which may be performed to help confirm biliary atresia include a biliary ultrasound scan, a HIDA scan and a percutaneous liver biopsy.

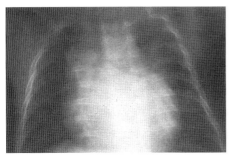

Fig 3.16.A

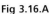

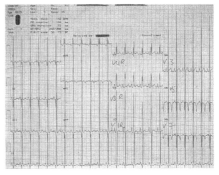

Fig 3.16.B

A 16-week-old boy was seen by a paediatrician after paucity of limb movement was noted at an 8-week check. Pregnancy and birth were uncomplicated; no problems were noted. Feeding was difficult and slow. Examination showed the boy to be strikingly floppy, lying in frog-leg posture, with little spontaneous movement (he could move his limbs against gravity); marked head lag was noted, his mouth hung open with tongue protruding. Liver was 1 cm enlarged. Chest and cardiovascular examination appeared clinically normal. CXR and ECG are shown. Other tests were as follows: CK 1282 units/l; AST 426 units/l; CKMB 40 units/l; CKMB/CK ratio 3%.

a. Describe the abnormalities in the electrocardiogram
   SELECT THE *THREE* MOST APPROPRIATE ANSWERS
   i. Superior axis deviation
   ii. Right atrial hypertrophy
   iii. Biventricular hypertrophy
   iv. First degree heart block
   v. ST depression
   vi. Inferior axis
   vii. Prolonged QT
   viii. Reverse RSR'

b. What further investigations are needed?
   SELECT THE *TWO* MOST APPROPRIATE ANSWERS
   i. Muscle biopsy
   ii. Echocardiogram
   iii. EEG
   iv. CSF for oligoclonal bands
   v. White cell enzyme assays

c. What is the likely diagnosis?
   SELECT *ONE* ANSWER
   i. Hypertrophic obstructive cardiomyopathy
   ii. Mucopolysaccharidosis
   iii. Glycogen storage disease type II (Pompe's disease)
   iv. Acute demyelinating encephalomyelitis
   v. Spinal muscular atrophy
   vi. Gaucher's disease

ANSWERS TO CASE 3.16

a. ii. Right atrial hypertrophy
    iii. Biventricular hypertrophy
    vi. Inferior axis
b. ii. Echocardiogram
    v. White cell enzyme assays
c. iii. Glycogen storage disease type II (Pompe's disease)

The CK is very high (normal range is up to 195 units/l). CKMB is also marginally raised (normal range is up to 25 units/l). CKMB/CK ratio is within normal range (normal range is up to 6%) indicating that the very high CK level is mainly of skeletal muscle origin.

Further investigations should include an echocardiogram and white cell enzyme assays.

The diagnosis is glycogen storage disease type-II (Pompe's disease, infantile acid maltase deficiency). Children with Pompe's disease usually die within the first 2 years of life due to rapidly progressing cardiomyopathy or aspiration pneumonia leading to cardio-respiratory failure.

Glycogen storage disease type-II is an autosomal recessive condition and, in the infantile variety (Pompe's disease), there is deficiency of a lysosomal enzyme 1,4 alpha-glucosidase. It characteristically presents in the first month of life with profound hypotonia, massive cardiomegaly, hyporeflexia and macroglossia. In this child, 1,4 alpha-glucosidase was found to be very deficient, confirming the suspicion of Pompe's disease.

Physical signs in Pompe's disease include: hypotonia, progressive weakness, absent reflexes, hepatomegaly and cardiomegaly.

Fifteen-year-old John developed a sore throat on a school skiing holiday in Switzerland. He had also had a sore throat 2 months before. On returning to the UK, a widespread non-itchy rash appeared. The day before, he had had a little neck stiffness which had totally resolved overnight. John's best friend had the same problems during the holiday.

John's temperature was 36°C. Heart rate and blood pressure were normal. The rash was pink, macular and blanching. His tonsils appeared reddened. The rest of his examination was normal.

John was asked to return 2 days later for review. The rash had spread further, but did not involve his face. Otherwise, he was entirely well, afebrile and the rest of his examination was again normal. Results from the initial presentation were: Hb 12.8 g/dl, WBC 28×10^9/l, neutrophils 25.2×10^9/l, platelets 272×10^9/l, CRP 243 mg/l, Monospot negative. The throat swab had disappeared.

Blood tests were repeated.

The health authority contacted the family, as another child from the school skiing holiday had been hospitalised with meningococcal disease. John was given prophylaxis, and returned to the hospital. The rash remained, but he was well. The repeat blood tests had shown Hb 12.6 g/dl, WBC 9.6×10^9/l, platelets 411×10^9/l, CRP 54 mg/l. On this third visit, further repetition showed Hb 12.4×10^9/l, WBC 9.4×10^9/l, platelets 511×10^9/l, CRP 4 mg/l.

He and his parents are frightened: could it be meningitis?

What do you say?

SELECT THE *THREE* BEST ANSWERS

  i. It is likely that John has glandular fever
 ii. It is possible that John has meningococcal disease
iii. It is unlikely that John has meningococcal disease
 iv. It is unlikely that John has glandular fever
  v. It is possible that John has meningitis
 vi. The symptomatology is too mild for untreated meningococcal disease
vii. Meningococcal disease always presents acutely
viii. John possibly needs treatment with antibiotics

ANSWERS TO CASE 3.17

ii. It is possible that John has meningococcal disease
iv. It is unlikely that John has glandular fever
viii. John possibly needs treatment with antibiotics

Repeated clinical examination has not shown meningism. It is very unlikely that John has meningitis. Meningococcal disease can present as meningitis and/or septicaemia. Septicaemia usually presents acutely with rapid onset and fatality. The classic rash is petechial and/or purpuric. However, there is also a subacute form, which may also have generalized petechial rash and may progress to cause focal infection in the meninges, joints, heart or eye. The chronic form of meningococcal sepsis may have anorexia, weight loss, fever, arthralgia or arthritis and a non-itchy, blanching, macular skin rash. Erythema nodosum or bacterial endocarditis may occur.

In its early stages, even the acute form of meningococcal disease, soon to fulminate, may have a macular, blanching or even urticarial rash.

The differential diagnosis of meningococcaemia may be broad. A morbilliform rash may be caused by a drug or other allergy, or viral infections including measles. Other bacterial and viral infections may cause purpura. Henoch–Schonlein disease usually has purpura, but may be macular. Idiopathic thrombocytopaenic purpura gives petechiae, purpura or bruising.

Subacute and chronic meningococcaemia present additional challenges, with a differential diagnosis including many causes of arthritis and fever.

Further tests include blood for culture, PCR and serology. Swab from posterior pharyngeal wall (either orally or per nasally). A scrape of the rash may show meningococci.

John's tests showed that he had meningococcaemia. Treated with antibiotics, he suffered no ill effects.

CASE 3.18

1. Coeliac disease
2. Crohn's disease
3. Ulcerative colitis
4. Cows' milk protein intolerance
5. Toddlers' diarrhoea
6. Cystic fibrosis
7. Lactose intolerance
8. Irritable bowel syndrome
9. Abdominal migraine
10. Haemolytic uraemic syndrome (HUS)

For each of the following case scenarios select the most likely diagnosis from the list above.

a. A-15-year old boy presents with delayed puberty and short stature. Both parents' height lies on the 75th centile. He looks pale and thin. He recently presented to his general practitioner with a painful red swelling on his shin which has now resolved. Examination reveals aphthous ulceration in his mouth, but is otherwise unremarkable.

b. A 3-year-old has intermittent diarrhoea with stools of varying consistency and sometimes undigested food particles. His growth is following the 9th centile. His mother is concerned and has tried to reduce his intake of dairy produce but his symptoms have not improved.

c. An 11-month-old infant presents with a history of persistent loose stools and poor weight gain since breast feeding was discontinued at 9 months. He has had antibiotics on two occasions from his general practitioner for chest infections. Initial investigations reveal a mild metabolic alkalosis with hypokalaemia.

a. 2. Crohn's disease

Crohn's is a chronic granulomatous inflammatory disease of the bowel involving the whole gastrointestinal tract from mouth to anus. The inflammation is transmural with skip lesions. Presenting symptoms include abdominal pain, diarrhoea and weight loss, although there may be no abdominal symptoms. Growth failure with delayed bone maturation and delayed puberty can occur. There has been an increase in the incidence of Crohn's over the last few years.

b. 5. Toddlers' diarrhoea

This is a clinical syndrome characterised by chronic diarrhoea often with undigested food in the stools of a child who is otherwise well, gaining weight and growing satisfactorily. Bowels may be opened up to six times a day, and stools may contain mucus (but no blood). Stools are often looser towards the end of the day. Symptoms usually start between 8 and 20 months of age, and there may be a family history of irritable bowel syndrome. No treatment other than reassurance is necessary.

c. 6. Cystic fibrosis

CF is a multisystem disease and is characterised by the production of very viscous mucus at epithelial surfaces. Inheritance is autosomal recessive and prevalence is $1:2000$, with a carrier frequency of $1:20$. There is a deletion on the long arm of chromosome 7, which results in a defect in a transmembrane regulator protein called the cystic fibrosis transmembrane conductance regulator (CFTR). This represents a cAMP mediated chloride channel. In the lungs, normal CFTR causes efflux of chloride ions across apical membranes of the submucosal glands, followed by sodium and water. In CF, there is an inability to secrete chloride, sodium and water, resulting in thick secretions. A similar problem occurs in the pancreatic and biliary ducts. However, in the skin, the function of sweat glands is to absorb chloride from the isotonic sweat, so in CF, this doesn't happen and there is therefore a high sweat chloride and sodium (the basis of the sweat test).

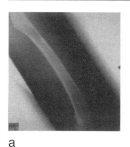
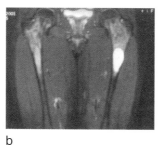
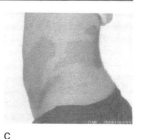

a   b   c

Fig 3.19

A 10-year-old girl complained of pain in her upper left thigh since the age of 7 years, which had been attributed to growing pains. However, the pain had persisted and recently got worse requiring analgesia. Plain X-ray (Fig. 3.19.a) showed an abnormality, which was imaged by MRI (Fig.3.19.b). Physical examination revealed her as having three large café au lait marks which had been present since birth (Fig. 3.19.c). She was pubertal at Tanner breast stage 4. Whole-body radionucleotide scanning revealed multiple bony abnormalities which were asymptomatic. Bone biochemistry and gonadotrophin releasing hormone stimulation tests results are shown:

Table 3.19.1

Ca (2.1-2.6) mmol/l	PO₄ (0.9-1.8) mmol/l	ALP (150-570) IU/l	TRP (>80%)	TmPO₄/ GFR	Peak LH IU/l (1.4-2.6)	Peak FSH IU/l	Oestradiol (75-1470) pmol/l
2.43	0.92	1406	87%	0.8	10.9	7.2	78

TRP: tubular reabsorption of phosphate; TmPO₄/GFR: tubular reabsorption of phosphate corrected for glomerular filtration rate, numbers in brackets indicate normal ranges

What is the likely diagnosis?

SELECT *ONE* ANSWER ONLY
  i. McCune Albright syndrome
 ii. Osteomalacia
iii. Fanconi syndrome
iv. Neurofibromatosis type I
 v. Ollier's disease
vi. Osteopetrosis

ANSWER TO CASE 3.19

i. McCune Albright syndrome

The likely diagnosis is McCune Albright syndrome. However, characteristically, MAS is associated with skin lesions, bony lesions and endocrinopathies.

The plain X-ray shows a bone cyst in the femur, which is confirmed in the MRI scan in the left upper thigh and the skin pigmentation in Figure 3.19.1c shows coast of Maine pigmented café au lait spots. The multiple asymptomatic bony abnormalities revealed on the radionucleotide scan demonstrate polyostotic fibrous dysplasia.

The most common associated endocrinopathy is gonadotrophin-independent precocious puberty where luteinised follicular cysts within the ovaries function autonomously. Pituitary adenomas capable of secreting excess LH, FSH, GH and/or prolactin have been reported. Patients may have Cushing's syndrome and hyperthyroidism due to autonomous multinodular hyperplasia. The syndrome occurs in incomplete as well as in expanded forms. Precocious puberty and bone lesions may occur in the absence of cutaneous manifestations; furthermore, not all patients have sexual precocity. This patient has an early puberty since she is at Tanner breast stage 4 at an age of 10.3 years. Her GnRH stimulation tests demonstrate a centrally mediated pubertal response, in keeping with normal centrally mediated puberty.

Renal phosphate wasting may occur in MAS, resulting in hypophosphataemic rickets. Calcium and phosphate are often normal but alkaline phosphatase and other biochemical markers of bone turnover may be elevated as in this case where phosphorus is at the lower end of normal range with raised alkaline phospatase and low TmPO4 when corrected for GFR. These patients may benefit from treatment with phosphate supplements and a vitamin D analogue. Recently, the bisphosphonate, pamidronate, given i.v. has been used for bone pain.

Chapter 4

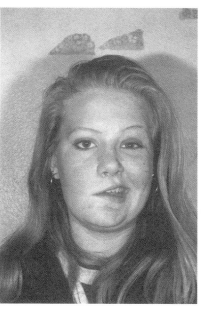

(1) Bells palsy (LMNL)
(2) Ramsey Hunt (Herpetic)
(3) Mobeius Synd. 6th nv psy

Fig 4.1

What are the three most important signs to elicit during examination of this 16 year-old girl?

SELECT *THREE* ANSWERS ONLY
  i. Trigeminal nerve paraesthesia
 ii. Tenderness over temporal region
iii. Involvement of frontalis muscle
 iv. Associated herpetic lesions in the external auditory meatus
  v. Pupillary constriction
 vi. Associated hearing impairment

ANSWERS TO CASE 4.1

iii. Involvement of frontalis muscle
iv. Associated herpetic lesions in the external auditory meatus
vi. Associated hearing impairment

This girl has right-sided facial nerve palsy. The differential diagnosis includes Bell's palsy, Moebius syndrome and Ramsay–Hunt syndrome.

It is important to establish the following during your examination:
Whether it is an upper or lower motor neurone deficit (Bell's palsy is a lower motor neurone lesion – thus the forehead is involved)
Associated herpetic vesicles in the external auditory meatus (Ramsay–Hunt)
Associated VI nerve palsy (possibly Moebius syndrome but usually bilateral)
Associated hearing impairment (possible acoustic neuroma)
Can the patient close the eyelids? (indication for methylcellulose eyedrops)

Facial nerve

In supranuclear paralysis (upper motor neurone) only the lower part of the face is involved because of the bilateral upper motor neurone innervation of the forehead. In infranuclear paralysis (lower motor neurone), both the upper and lower parts of the face are involved equally, e.g. Bell's palsy.

Patterns of muscular weakness

- Upper motor neurone: increased tone, increased reflexes, pyramidal pattern of weakness (weak extensors in the arm, weak flexors in the legs)
- Lower motor neurone: wasting, fasciculation, decreased tone and absent reflexes

CASE 4.2

A full-term infant was delivered by emergency Caesarean section for placental abruption. Immediately before the Caesarean section, there had been a fetal bradycardia. At delivery, he was white, bradycardic and made no respiratory effort. He required bag and mask ventilation for the first 12 min of life following which he started to gasp and breathe normally. His Apgar scores were 1 at 1 min and 5 at 5 min. The cord pH was 6.85. After admission to the neonatal unit, he remained lethargic and hypotonic. The initial arterial blood gas showed the following:

pH 6.95
PCO_2 2.6 kPa
PO_2 11.3 kPa
HCO_3 14 mmol/l
Base excess −20 mmol/l
Lactate 15.4 mmol/l

A cranial ultrasound scan was normal. His condition improved, although he required oro-gastric tube feeds until 6 days old, following which he started to feed normally by bottle. At discharge, neurological examination was normal.

a. Which of the following is not an expected complication during the neonatal period?
SELECT *ONE* ANSWER ONLY
  i. Hepatic necrosis
  ii. Seizures
  iii. Renal dysfunction
  iv. Hypertension
  v. Deranged coagulation
  vi. Hyaline membrane disease

b. Which clinical factors suggest a worse prognosis?
SELECT *THREE* ANSWERS ONLY
  i. Hypothermia
  ii. Hypertonia
  iii. Irritability
  iv. Prematurity
  v. Severe hypotonia
  vi. Seizures
  vii. Unconsciousness

ANSWERS TO CASE 4.2

a. iv. Hypertension
b. v. Severe hypotonia
    vi. Seizures
    vii. Unconsciousness

This baby has hypoxic–ischaemic encephalopathy (HIE). Complications include renal failure, hepatic necrosis (elevated liver enzymes), clotting abnormalities and DIC, hyaline membrane disease, persistent pulmonary hypertension, and myocardial dysfunction (hypotension, low cardiac output).

Clinical assessment of this condition is the most useful way to assess severity and prognosis. Sarnat and Sarnat described the clinical grading of HIE. There are three grades of severity recognised.

Grade I: Irritability, hypotonia, increased arousal, poor feeding initially but improving by day 2-3. No seizures. Good outcome usual (<2% have severe handicap).

Grade II: Lethargy, abnormal tone, may be some multi-organ involvement (renal failure, hepatic impairment, etc.). Seizures. Poor feeding for first week of life. Variable outcome.

Grade III: Multi-organ involvement, decreased consciousness level or unconsciousness, severe hypotonia, prolonged and difficult to control seizures. Death or poor outcome very likely (70-80%).

The neurological behaviour during the neonatal period remains the best prognostic marker. This infant had a Sarnat grade II hypoxic ischaemic encephalopathy. Approximately 20% of infants with HIE of this severity will have developmental impairment. The poor prognostic features in this case are that the first gasp was at 12 min of age, the infant had seizures, the cord and arterial pH were both low (<7.0) and the lactate (and base excess) was high. The good prognostic features were that he responded to anticonvulsants and did not continue to fit, had a normal neurological examination before discharge, and bottle fed within a week of age. The normal cranial ultrasound scan does not help to guide prognosis. Imaging using CT or MRI may be useful particularly if performed after the first week of life, and EEG has also been shown to predict outcome. There are no clinical interventions which have been shown to improve outcome, but there has been recent interest in the use of hypothermia as a therapeutic manoeuvre.

CASE 4.3

A male infant was born at 38 weeks' gestation, by spontaneous vertex delivery, weighing 4500 g. You are asked to see the baby in the postnatal ward at 48 h of age because the mother feels he has a large tongue. On examination he is settled and sleeping. He has a large and slightly protruding tongue, linear creases on both ear lobes and an umbilical hernia. Examination of his abdomen reveals 2 cm of liver palpable but is otherwise normal.

a. What investigation would you carry out first?
    SELECT *ONE* ANSWER ONLY
    i. Ultrasound abdomen
    ii. Serum calcium
    iii. Echocardiogram
    iv. Check patency of oesophagus with nasogastric tube
    v. Blood glucose
    vi. Examination of palate

b. What condition is the baby at risk of in later life?
    SELECT *ONE* ANSWER ONLY
    i. Leukaemia
    ii. Coeliac disease
    iii. Wilm's tumour
    iv. Diabetes mellitus
    v. Eisenmenger's syndrome
    vi. Glue ear
    vii. Osteoporosis

ANSWERS TO CASE 4.3

a. v. Blood glucose
b. iii. Wilm's tumour

This baby has several features which suggest Beckwith–Wiedemann syndrome: macrosomia, macroglossia, ear lobe creases and an umbilical hernia.

Congenital hypothyroidism, which could give you macroglossia and umbilical hernia, would not result in macrosomia or the characteristic ear lobe creases.

Beckwith–Wiedemann syndrome is related to an abnormality in the chromosome 11p15.5 region. Other features include mild microcephaly, hemihypertrophy, neonatal polycythaemia and cryptorchidism. Omphalocoele/exomphalos or other umbilical anomalies may be present. Babies may have feeding and associated breathing problems in the neonatal period related to size of tongue.

Mild-to-moderate mental deficiency present in some cases is related to undiagnosed and/or untreated hypoglycaemia that is present in 33-50% of cases. Otherwise, mental function appears to be normal.

Children with Beckwith–Wiedemann are at risk of developing tumours, in particular Wilm's tumour, hepatoblastoma, adrenal carcinoma and gonadoblastoma.

CASE 4.4

MRCPCH Part 2

A 10-year-old boy presents with a 3-month history of gradually increasing weakness, lassitude, dizziness and some abdominal pain. His schoolwork has deteriorated a little. On examination he is found to be hypotensive and collapses on standing. Basic serum biochemistry shows:

Urea 5 mmol/l
Creatinine 80 μmol/l
Na 127 mmol/l
K 5.8 mmol/l
Ca 2.3 mmol/l

a. What findings on examination may prove helpful?
    SELECT *TWO* ANSWERS ONLY
  i. Acanthosis nigrans
 ii. Buccal mucosa pigmentation
iii. Ejection systolic murmur
 iv. Cataracts
  v. Pigmented scars
 vi. Eczema

b. What other investigations would you consider?
    SELECT *THREE* ANSWERS ONLY
   i. Adrenal antibodies
  ii. Glucagon stimulation test
 iii. Testosterone
  iv. ACTH stimulation test
   v. Adrenal USS
  vi. CT head
 vii. 17-hydroxyprogesterone
viii. Echocardiogram
  ix. Karyotype

ANSWERS TO CASE 4.4

a. ii. Buccal mucosa pigmentation
    v. Pigmented scars
c.   i. Adrenal antibodies
    iv. ACTH stimulation test
    v. Adrenal USS

The findings of hyponatraemia, hyperkalaemia and hypoglycaemia point to a diagnosis of Addison's disease. The finding of hyperpigmentation on examination would be helpful in making the diagnosis. Such increased pigmentation often has the appearance of a well suntanned skin; freckles and old scars may darken and there is also sometimes pigmenting of the buccal mucosa.

Further investigations should include an ACTH stimulation test, adrenal antibodies (e.g. antiadrenal cytoplasmic antibody) are usually raised, and screening for other autoantibody disorders that may occur with Addison's (e.g. diabetes mellitus and hypoparathyroidism). In the majority of cases Addison's is an autoimmune disorder but very long chain fatty acids should be requested in this boy as there is an association with adrenoleukodystrophy and he is having difficulties at school. Imaging of the adrenal glands may prove useful in identifying other more rare causes.

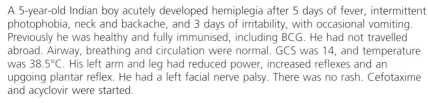
A 5-year-old Indian boy acutely developed hemiplegia after 5 days of fever, intermittent photophobia, neck and backache, and 3 days of irritability, with occasional vomiting. Previously he was healthy and fully immunised, including BCG. He had not travelled abroad. Airway, breathing and circulation were normal. GCS was 14, and temperature was 38.5°C. His left arm and leg had reduced power, increased reflexes and an upgoing plantar reflex. He had a left facial nerve palsy. There was no rash. Cefotaxime and acyclovir were started.

CT head showed no space-occupying lesion, no signs of raised intracranial pressure, but meningeal enhancement with contrast. In 8 h, his neurological deficits had greatly improved. After careful consideration, a lumbar puncture was performed.

Blood results were: Hb 11.3 g/dl, WBC 15.6 × 10^9/l, neutrophils 11.3 × 10^9/l, platelets 207 × 10^9/l, CRP 80 mg/l, Na 128 mmol/l, K 3.4 mmol/l, urea 5.3 mmol/l, creatinine 57 mmol/l, Ca 2.21 mmol/l and glucose 7.8 mmol/l.

CSF results were: glucose <0.6 mmol/l, lactate 10.4 mmol/l, protein 0.95 g/l, WBC 500/mm^3 (99% lymphocytes), red blood cells 45/mm^3, no organisms seen.

Which of the following is the most likely diagnosis?

SELECT *ONE* ANSWER ONLY

   i. Viral meningitis
  ii. Tuberculosis
 iii. Listeria
 iv. Cryptococcus
  v. Acute bacterial meningitis

PASS

ANSWER TO CASE 4.5

iii. Listeria

The differential diagnosis includes tuberculosis, listeria, cryptococcus, and acute bacterial meningitis (which can present with lymphocytic infiltrate). Although viral meningitis is possible, it is unlikely as the CSF glucose is very low.

Following the CSF results, antituberculous chemotherapy (rifampicin, isoniazid and pyrazinamide) should be added, and either meropenem or ampicillin to cover listeria. Steroids (for tuberculous meningitis with nerve palsies) and antifungals should be considered. Further investigations include:

For tuberculosis – Ziehl–Nielsen or auramine stain, CXR and tuberculin skin test
For cryptococcus – Indian ink stain and antigen tests

His CSF grew Gram-positive rods (Listeria monocytogenes). Ampicillin and gentamicin were given for synergy.

Listeria, an uncommon pathogen in the general population, is important in pregnancy, neonates, the elderly and those immunocompromised. In the USA, incidence is 7.4 cases per million population: 27% being pregnant women. Seventy per cent of non-perinatal infections are in immunocompromised patients. Lower incidence figures have been reported in the UK. No impairment of the host defences of this child has been found. Contaminated food is usually the source. Listeria has been isolated from raw meat, dairy products (particularly soft cheeses and unpasteurised milk), vegetables and seafood. No source of infection for this child was identified.

The most common manifestation is diarrhoea. Fever, nausea, vomiting and diarrhoea may resemble gastrointestinal illness. Recently, it has been associated with epidemic gastroenteritis. Bacteraemia and meningitis are more serious. Listeria has a predilection for the brain parenchyma, especially the brain stem and the meninges. Mental status changes are common. Seizures occur in at least 25%. Cranial nerve deficits may be present. Neck stiffness is less common. Movement disorders may include tremor, myoclonus and ataxia. There may be encephalitis, particularly brain stem. Brain abscess occurs in 10% of CNS infections and has high mortality. Blood cultures are positive in 60-75% of patients with CNS infections. Listeria demonstrates 'tumbling motility' in wet mounts of CSF. CSF Gram stain is positive in 50%, and culture in nearly 100%. Serologic testing is unreliable.

Early-onset neonatal listeriosis has a 20-30% mortality rate. Late-onset neonatal listeriosis has a 0-20% mortality rate. Mortality in older children is less than 10%. Hydrocephalus, mental retardation and other CNS sequelae have been reported in survivors of Listeria meningitis.

CASE 4.6

A 3-week-old ex-29-week infant remained in the neonatal unit nursery for nasogastric feeding, monitoring of apnoea and bradycardia, and treatment of gastro-oesophageal reflux with ranitidine and cisapride. Erythromycin was commenced for what was thought to be a mild atypical pneumonia. Twelve hours later this infant had an unexpected cardiac arrest just before a feed and died.

Echocardiogram during attempted resuscitation showed ventricular fibrillation. Post-mortem showed no milk in the trachea.

A resting ECG taken the previous week had shown HR 150/minute; RR interval = 0.4 s; QT = 0.32 s.

a. What abnormality is demonstrated by the ECG?
   SELECT *ONE* ANSWER ONLY
   i. Tachycardia
   ii. Short RR
   iii. Long QT
   iv. Short QT
   v. Sinus arrhythmia

b. What are the likely factors contributing to the fatal episode?
   SELECT *TWO* ANSWERS ONLY
   i. Prematurity
   ii. Cisapride treatment
   iii. Nasogastric feeding
   iv. Erythromycin therapy
   v. Associated apnoea

ANSWERS TO CASE 4.6

a. iii. Long QT
b. ii. Cisapride treatment
    iv. Erythromycin therapy

These results show prolonged QT syndrome. The corrected QT interval is calculated by

$$QTc = \frac{QT}{\sqrt{RR}}$$

The upper normal limit of QTc: 0.45 s for boys; 0.46 s for girls. In this case the QTc is 0.51 s.

The QT prolongation is probably secondary to cisapride and exacerbated by erythromycin. Prolonged QT can also be exacerbated by hypocalcaemia.

Cisapride is no longer used for the routine treatment of reflux, although it can be prescribed in rare circumstances, when a resting ECG must be performed first. Other drugs which can precipitate prolongation of the QT include:
   macrolides
   antihistamines
   salbutamol

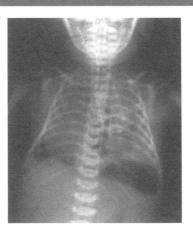

Fig 4.7

This term newborn baby developed respiratory difficulties shortly after birth. There were diminished air sounds bilaterally but particularly on the left side. The apex beat was located on the right, there were no murmurs and the pulses were all easily palpable. The abdominal examination was normal.

a. What is the diagnosis?
    SELECT THE *BEST* ANSWER
  i. CCAML
  ii. Congenital diaphragmatic hernia
  iii. Congenital pneumonia
  iv. Bilateral pneumothoraces
  v. Staphylococcal pneumatocoeles
  vi. Pulmonary interstitial emphysema

b. What would be your immediate management?
    SELECT THE *THREE* MOST APPROPRIATE ANSWERS
  i. Check blood gas and ventilate if necessary
  ii. Book emergency theatre
  iii. Paralyse
  iv. Urgent echo to exclude associated cardiac lesion
  v. Intubate and ventilate
  vi. Sedate

ANSWERS TO CASE 4.7

a. ii. Congenital diaphragmatic hernia
b. iii. Paralyse
   v. Intubate and ventilate
   vi. Sedate

The CXR shows bowel gas shadowing, most visible at the mediastinum and the left chest. This is a diaphragmatic hernia. A scaphoid abdomen is not necessarily a feature.

A number of different diaphragmatic hernias have been described. Retrosternal (Morgagni) and posterolateral (Bochdalek) are the two classical defects. At 8 weeks' gestation the pleuroperitoneal canals close, separating the abdominal and thoracic cavities. Failure of these canals to close may be just one cause. Other mechanisms, such as disruption of the developing thoracic mesenchyme, have been postulated.

Sedation, paralysis, ventilation and nasogastric drainage are generally the most important initial management steps. In utero reduction is being attempted in certain centres.

A 14-month-old girl was brought into accident and emergency (A&E) by ambulance at 0600 h one morning, fitting. Her parents gave a history that she had been well until the previous morning when she had developed a coryzal illness. She had been seen by the GP, who noted that she was pyrexial and diagnosed a viral illness. She had fed poorly that day, had been drowsy and had been vomiting. She had gone to bed without eating, although she had tolerated some clear fluid. She slept in her parents' bed that night and they were woken by her fitting. Her parents were healthy and unrelated. There was no family history of note; she was their first child.

On arrival in A&E, she was still fitting. She had a temperature of 38.5°C but no rash. She had hepatomegaly. Her initial investigations showed:

Na 129 mmol/l	K 4.4 mmol/l
Urea 3.7 mmol/l	Creatinine 55 μmol/l
Glucose 0.9 mmol/l	
AST 256 u/l	ALP 350 u/l
Bilirubin 30 μmol/l	Ammonia 88 μmol/l (10-47)

Urine dipstick negative, no ketones

a. What would your initial management be?
   SELECT *THREE* ANSWERS ONLY
   i. 100% oxygen
   ii. Phenobarbitone
   iii. i.v. glucose infusion 6-8 mg/kg/min
   iv. Sodium benzoate
   v. Bolus of iv glucose
   vi. 0.9% NaCl infusion
   vii. i.v. lorazepam

b. What is the likely diagnosis?
   SELECT *ONE* ANSWER ONLY
   i. Hyponatraemic seizures
   ii. Meningococcaemia
   iii. Diabetes insipidus
   iv. Medium-chain acyl-CoA dehydrogenase deficiency

ANSWERS TO CASE 4.8

a. i. 100% oxygen
    v. Bolus of i.v. dextrose
    vii. i.v. lorazepam
b. iv. Medium chain acyl-CoA dehydrogenase (MCAD) deficiency

Initial management involves care of the airway and breathing, and administering 100% oxygen. Appropriate blood specimens should be taken and a bolus of i.v. 10% glucose 2-5 ml/kg given followed by a continuous infusion providing 6-8 mg/kg/min glucose. Seizures should be treated according to the status epilepticus protocol. The glucose should be rechecked after 3-4 min and a repeat glucose bolus given if still <4 mmol/l.

Bloods should be obtained at the time of hypoglycaemia without delaying treatment. Samples to be sent immediately should include: glucose, lactate, ammonia, U&Es, LFT, FBC, CRP, blood cultures and blood gas. Samples should be immediately frozen and stored for: plasma amino acids, cortisol, GH, ACTH, ketone bodies, free fatty acids, medium chain fatty acids, carnitine, uric acid, triglycerides. Blood spots should be sent for acylcarnitine. The first urine voided (catheterise if necessary) is vital, and should be sent for ketones, reducing substances, organic and amino acids and toxicology.

There is no typical presentation of MCAD deficiency, but children often present between 3 and 15 months of age with an episode of vomiting and lethargy following a period of fasting. There may be an associated minor illness. In 20% of families, there may be a history of unexplained sibling deaths. The initial laboratory findings are of hypoglycaemia (although normal blood glucose levels have been seen), mild elevation of ammonia (50-100 μmol/l), mild elevation of transaminases, and hypoketosis.

CASE 4.9

A 10-year-old boy presents with a history of nervous twitches from the age of 4 years, which vary over time and fluctuate in severity. Mouth opening, eye blinking, grimacing and arching of his neck have been witnessed. He compulsively clears his throat and makes grunting noises. The problems are worse when he is under stress. His behaviour in school is problematic but parental management seems appropriate. He is attention seeking and impulsive, cannot wait his turn and shouts out in class. He is fidgety and frequently gets out of his seat. His concentration is poor in class, yet he performs well when working alone. Background knowledge and verbal performance are good but his educational progress has slowed. He is described as moody but well behaved at home. He enjoys drawing and is meticulous. His parents are concerned about his social adjustment. Birth and medical history are unremarkable. The parents are healthy and did not experience similar difficulties. A distant relative has epilepsy and a grandparent has Parkinson's disease. Examination including neurological assessment is normal. Involuntary twitches are witnessed, although there is no dystonia or choreiform movement. An EEG has been reported to be normal with movement artefact.

What is the most likely diagnosis?

SELECT *ONE* ANSWER ONLY

  i. Tourette's syndrome
 ii. Accidental ingestion
iii. Parkinsonism
 iv. Wilson's disease
  v. Obsessive-compulsive disorder
 vi. Post-streptococcal neuropsychiatric disorder
vii. Carbon monoxide encephalopathy

ANSWER TO CASE 4.9

i. Tourette's syndrome (TS)

Tourette's syndrome is a neuropsychiatric disorder of childhood onset. Diagnostic criteria include multiple (two or more) motor tics, at least one vocal tic, and duration of symptoms longer than 1 year. Prevalence is ~1–3% in children, higher in boys. Peak onset is at 5–7 years. Motor or vocal tics may be simple (e.g. shrugs, grimaces, barks and grunts) or complex (e.g. smelling, touching, copropraxia, coprolalia and echolalia). Flamboyant phenomena are rare. Tourette's syndrome has also been reported secondary to lamotrogine medication, in citrullinaemia, perinatal asphyxia, Down's syndrome and autism.

Differential diagnoses include:

- basal ganglia disorders, e.g. Wilson's disease, carbon monoxide encephalopathy, post-encephalitic parkinsonism and tardive dyskinesia (unlikely in this case)
- accidental ingestion or deliberate poisoning (acute presentation)
- PANDAS (Paediatric autoimmune neuropsychiatric disorders associated with streptococcal infection) – infection-triggered, autoimmune subtype of paediatric obsessive compulsive disorder and Tourette's syndrome – the working criteria include presence of OCD and/or tic disorder, prepubertal onset, acute presentation, episodic symptom severity, recent group A beta-haemolytic streptococcal infection and neurological abnormalities

If the presentation is typical and careful neurological evaluation is normal, no further investigations are indicated. Investigations may be indicated in atypical cases. The EEG is non-specific in Tourette's syndrome. Radiological investigations are unlikely to be informative.

Associated conditions include OCD, ADD/H, specific learning problems, visuomotor difficulties and migraine (more prevalent in Tourette's syndrome). Comorbid disorders are often more detrimental than the tics. The ADD/H child may be perceived as deliberately naughty or disruptive. Obsessional behaviour may bring the child into conflict with others. The child may experience low self-esteem, anxiety and depression, teasing and bullying. School difficulties might therefore be related to educational problems, psychopathology, use of tic-suppressing medication or the direct consequences of having a stigmatising condition.

The goal of management is to plan individualised therapy to deal with the major causes of distress, comorbid conditions and complications. The family and those in the social and educational sphere need information. Specialist involvement may be required. Medication may be used to reduce tics, control obsessive-compulsive behaviour or attention problems, or to treat anxiety and depression. Drugs that suppress tics block dopamine and noradrenaline receptors, e.g. haloperidol, pimozide and sulpiride. Acetylcholine-blocking or dopamine-releasing agents may be used for ADD/H, e.g. clonidine and methylphenidate (may exacerbate tics). Medication that blocks serotonin reuptake may help OCD and depression, e.g. tricyclic antidepressants and fluoxetine. No medication is ideal.

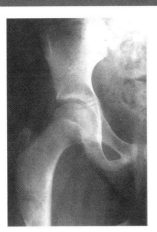

Fig 4.10

A 9-year old girl with known Von Willebrand's disease (VWD) presented with a 3-month history of right thigh and knee pain. There was no history of trauma. Other than VWD, there was no significant past medical history. On examination she was well. There was no fever and no rash. Systemic examination was entirely normal. On examination of her right leg, there were no signs of bruising or erythema. There was no swelling of any joints and she had a normal examination of her knee and ankle joints. On examination of her hip, external rotation was limited by pain but was otherwise normal. X-ray examination of her hips revealed a transverse fracture of the femoral shaft just below the level of the lesser trochanter.

a. What are the possible diagnoses?
   SELECT *TWO* ANSWERS ONLY
   i. Osteogenesis imperfecta
   ii. Primary bone tumour
   iii. Juvenile rheumatoid arthritis
   iv. Fibrous dysplasia
   v. Slipped upper femoral epiphysis

b. What investigations would you like to do?
   SELECT *TWO* ANSWERS ONLY
   i. αFP, HCG, CEA
   ii. CXR
   iii. Autoimmune screen
   iv. Fibroblast culture
   v. DEXA scan

ANSWERS TO CASE 4.10

a. ii. Primary bone tumour
    iv. Fibrous dysplasia
b. i. αFP, HCG, CEA
    ii. CXR

The most common reason for a pathological fracture in this age group is an isolated area of fibrous dysplasia, as in this case. It commonly presents in mid to late childhood. The areas of fibrous dysplasia are benign and may be isolated or multiple (polyostotic). Polyostotic fibrous dysplasia associated with skin hyperpigmentation and endocrine dysfunction (commonly precocious puberty) is known as Albright's syndrome.

Primary malignancies may present with a pathological fracture, e.g. Ewing's sarcoma. Metastases from a distant primary malignancy (e.g. neuroblastoma, kidney, thyroid) should also be considered. Chronic bone infection is also a differential diagnosis. Appearances on X-ray are a helpful guide to diagnosis that may be further aided by MRI.

Investigations which may be necessary include FBC, U&E, LFT, CRP, Ca, and PO_4. Also αFP, HCG, CEA (as tumour markers), a CXR (to exclude mediastinal tumour), an abdominal USS (to look for evidence of neuroblastoma), urine HVA and VMA, an MRI of the lesion and a bone scan.

CASE 4.11

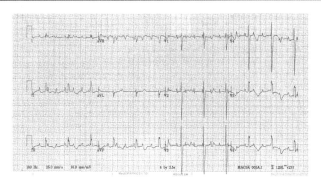

Fig 4.11

A pregnant woman was admitted at 32 weeks' gestation feeling unwell and vomiting. Her antenatal course had been uneventful prior to this admission, and the 20-week anomaly scan was reported as normal. Initial assessment revealed a fetal bradycardia, and the baby was delivered by emergency Caesarean section. At birth, the baby was blue with poor respiratory effort and a bradycardia of 60-70 bpm. She required intubation and ventilation which led to an improvement in colour but the heart rate remained below 100 bpm. On admission to the neonatal unit, a CXR revealed marked hyaline membrane disease, and an ECG was obtained.

a. What is the ECG abnormality?
   SELECT *ONE* ANSWER ONLY
   i. Short PR interval
   ii. Second degree heart block
   iii. Delayed repolarisation syndrome
   iv. Congenital complete heart block
   v. Prolonged QT interval

b. Which is the inotrope of choice in unstable babies with this condition?
   SELECT *ONE* ANSWER ONLY
   i. Dopamine
   ii. Noradrenaline
   iii. Isoprenaline
   iv. Atropine
   v. Flecainide

c. Which of the following maternal conditions can predispose to this condition?
   SELECT *ONE* ANSWER ONLY
   i. Parvovirus infection
   ii. Ehlers–Danlos syndrome
   iii. Sjögren's syndrome
   iv. Polyarteritis nodosa

ANSWERS TO CASE 4.11

a. iv. Congenital complete heart block (CCHB)
b. iii. Isoprenaline
c. iii. Sjögren's syndrome

The ECG shows congenital CHB which can be associated with a maternal history of systemic lupus erythematosus (SLE) or Sjögren's syndrome. The prevalence of congenital CHB in newborns of prospectively followed-up women already known to be anti-Ro/SSA positive and with known connective tissue disease is 2%. This finding is useful with regard to preconception counselling. The risk of delivering an infant with congenital CHB may be higher in mothers with Sjögren's syndrome than in those with SLE. Additional electrocardiographic abnormalities such as sinus bradycardia and prolongation of the QT interval may be present in their children.

An echocardiogram was carried out to exclude congenital heart disease. This baby had a large secundum atrial septal defect with bidirectional flow. The heart showed biventricular hypertrophy, presumably in response to longstanding heart block.

Pacing is the definitive management. The management of the preterm fetus with hydrops caused by congenital CHB is difficult, with associated morbidity and mortality.

CASE 4.12

A 7-year-old boy presented with an 18-month history of poor growth and failure to gain weight. His appetite was poor and he was lethargic such that he had to be carried home from school. There was no significant past medical history. On examination, he was pale and subdued. His weight and height were on the 0.4th percentile. He had a heart rate of 104/minute and a blood pressure of 128/65. There was a systolic murmur audible all over the praecordium.

Initial investigation showed:
Hb 4.5 g/dl
Na 141 mmol/l
K 4.4 mmol/l
Urea 80 mmol/l
Creatinine 907 µmol/l
Total Ca 1.23 mmol/l
Phosphate 3.19 mmol/l
Bicarbonate 8.7 mmol/l
PTH 248 pmol/l (0-7.3)
Urinalysis blood +, protein +

A working diagnosis of end-stage renal failure was made.

a. What non-haematological investigations would you like to perform?
SELECT *THREE* ANSWERS ONLY
   i. Echocardiography
   ii. Wrist X-ray
   iii. Chest X-ray
   iv. Bone marrow aspirate
   v. Renal ultrasound scan
   vi. 24 hour urinary protein collection
   vii. Parathyroid isotope scan

b. What are the effects of this condition which need to be addressed in the long-term management of this child?
SELECT *THREE* ANSWERS ONLY
   i. Risk of malignancy
   ii. Retinal degeneration
   iii. Nutrition and growth
   iv. Development of neuropathy
   v. Metabolic bone disease
   vi. Blood pressure
   vii. Psychosis

ANSWER TO CASE 4.12

a. i. Echocardiography
   ii. Wrist X-ray
   v. Renal ultrasound scan
b. iii. Nutrition and growth
   v. Metabolic bone disease
   vi. Blood pressure

The working diagnosis here is end-stage renal failure. This little boy has a GFR of less than 10 ml/min/1.73 m^2 and requires renal replacement therapy, i.e. dialysis. GFR = (height in cm × 40)/creatinine (μmol/l).

Investigations that need to be performed include a renal ultrasound scan to help establish the cause of the renal failure, an echocardiogram to determine the cause of the murmur, and the effect of the blood pressure, and a wrist X-ray should be done to confirm bone age and look for osteodystrophy.

The long-term management of this child includes careful fluid and electrolyte balance, maximising nutrition and growth, treating anaemia and metabolic bone disease, close observation of the blood pressure and psychological therapy.

CASE 4.13

A 5-year old girl presented for the third time in a year with peri-anal itching, particularly at night. A diagnosis of threadworm has been made by her GP in the past, and her mother reports having treated it with piperazine, following which her symptoms resolved on each occasion.

What is the likely cause for the child's illness?

SELECT *ONE* ANSWER ONLY

  i. *Ascaris lumbricoides*
 ii. *Ancylostoma duodenale*
 iii. *Sarcoptes scabiei*
 iv. *Wuchereria bancrofti*
  v. *Enterobius vermicularis* ⊚
 vi. *Ancylostoma braziliense*

ANSWER TO CASE 4.13

v. *Enterobius vermicularis*

This girl has recurrent *Enterobius vermicularis* infection, also known as threadworm or pinworm. Reinfection, and autoinfection (on the child's fingers following peri-anal scratching at night) are common.

Piperazine can be given as 2 doses 2 weeks apart, and the second dose may be missed, thus encouraging reinfection. Mebendazole or albendazole as a single dose is the first-line treatment. Recurrence despite adequate treatment is common.

Confirmation of the diagnosis can be made by the 'Sellotape' test, ideally taken in the morning before washing. The adhesive tape is applied to the peri-anal skin, where the eggs are laid, and applied to a slide to facilitate transport for examination under the microscope. It is possible to see the eggs using a magnifying glass oneself. The worms lay their eggs at night, and they may sometimes be seen on the peri-anal area at this time.

Threadworm may be carried by other members of the household, and treatment of all family members with a single dose of albendazole or mebendazole in this case would be indicated. Mebendazole is not recommended for children under 2 years, and 2 doses of piperazine 2 weeks apart is an alternative treatment. Finger nails should be kept short (to prevent eggs being trapped under the nail), and tight underwear at night may help prevent reinfection.

Complications are uncommon as tissue invasion does not occur. In girls, a vulvo-vaginitis is recognised, and may cause a vaginal discharge. Iron deficiency anaemia is not a complication, and if present is likely to be due to dietary or other causes. Although helminthiasis is often associated with eosinophilia, this is infrequently found in enterobius infections. Helminth infections have been associated with a reduced incidence of allergic diseases such as asthma.

No other investigations are necessary.

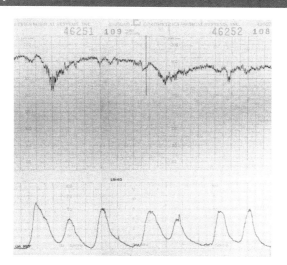

Fig 4.14

A woman expecting her first baby arrived at the delivery suite in established labour. Her temperature, pulse and blood pressure were within normal limits. The admission CTG was satisfactory, fetal movements were present and her membranes were intact. The following CTG was performed 4 h into the labour. The maternal pulse was 112 bpm and temperature 37.8°C.

a. Identify the principal features of this trace?
   SELECT THE *THREE* BEST ANSWERS
   i. Fetal bradycardia
   ii. Normal beat-to-beat variability
   iii. Type I decelerations
   iv. Late decelerations
   v. Flat trace
   vi. Fetal tachycardia
   vii. Reduced variability

b. Suggest reasons for a fetal tachycardia?
   SELECT THE *FIVE* BEST ANSWERS
   i. Maternal tachycardia
   ii. Fetal infection and pyrexia
   iii. Maternal infection
   iv. Maternal systemic lupus erythematosus (SLE)
   v. Preterm gestation
   vi. Post dates
   vii. Fetal cardiac anomaly
   viii. Maternal labetolol therapy
   ix. Developing fetal hypoxia

ANSWERS TO CASE 4.14

a. iv. Late decelerations
   vi. Fetal tachycardia
   vii. Reduced variability
b. ii. Fetal infection and pyrexia
   iii. Maternal infection
   v. Preterm gestation
   vii. Fetal cardiac anomaly
   ix. Developing fetal hypoxia

Fetal tachycardia is a baseline fetal heart rate >150 bpm. The fetal heart rate in this CTG is around 170-180 bpm. There is also reduced variability; normally the fetal heart rate varies over a minute between 10 to 25 bpm. When the variability is reduced, the rate varies between 6 and 10 bpm. A reduction in this variation is called a loss of baseline variability, and is associated with fetal hypoxia. Late decelerations are present on this CTG; these occur after the onset of the contraction. The greater the time lag after the onset of the contraction, the more sinister the trace.

Fetal tachycardia can be associated with any of the following: preterm gestation, developing fetal hypoxia, maternal anxiety and maternal pain, maternal dehydration, fetal activity, fetal infection and pyrexia, maternal infection and fetal cardiac anomaly.

Management of this case involves assessing the maternal condition and treating with i.v. antibiotics for presumed infection. A vaginal examination with artificial rupture of the membranes should be performed and the colour of the liquor assessed. Fetal blood sampling is useful to measure pH.

Close monitoring of the CTG and maternal progress is mandatory. The baby should be delivered immediately if fetal blood sampling shows a pH of <7.20 and the paediatrician should be present at delivery.

A 10-day-old male infant presented to the A&E department with a history of being found lifeless and floppy in his cot by his mother. On arrival at A&E, he was found to be apnoeic and bradycardic, with a capillary refill time of 6 s. He was intubated and fully resuscitated. Subsequent examination found the infant to be apyrexial and hypotonic, with widespread skin mottling but no other systemic abnormality. He subsequently had brief generalised seizures and was loaded with phenobarbitone. On making further enquiries into the history, it was noted that there had been a history of poor feeding for 24 h before presentation. The baby had been born at term in good condition and had been fully breast fed.

While he was being ventilated on the paediatric intensive therapy unit, it was noted that the baby had a mild persistent metabolic acidosis, and he continued to have seizures. He was extensively investigated.

Results included a raised valine level of 2900 µmol/l (normal 100-400 µmol/l), a leucine level of 2920 µmol/l (normal being 100-400 µmol/l) and an ammonia concentration of 142 µmol/l (normal 10-40 µmol/l).

a. What is the diagnosis?
   SELECT *ONE* ANSWER ONLY
   i. Pompé disease
   ii. Maple syrup urine disease
   iii. OTC deficiency
   iv. Methylmalonic acidaemia
   v. GM1-gangliosidosis
   vi. Galactosaemia

b. What is the most likely cause of the seizures?
   SELECT *ONE* ANSWER ONLY
   i. Associated hypoglycaemia
   ii. Hypocalcaemia
   iii. Raised leucine
   iv. Thiamine deficency
   v. Raised valine
   vi. Hyperammonaemia

ANSWERS TO CASE 4.15

a. ii. Maple syrup urine disease
b. iii. Raised leucine

With the initial history given, the three main differential diagnoses which must be considered are: (1) Neonatal sepsis. (2) Inborn error of metabolism. (3) Subdural haemorrhage.

Investigations that should be performed include:
- FBC and differential
- blood glucose
- U&Es
- LFTs
- Calcium, phosphate and magnesium
- blood gases
- full septic screen including CSF culture
- CXR
- cranial ultrasound
- CT head

The diagnosis here is maple syrup urine disease.

The seizures are caused by the very high levels of leucine and the ketoacids that result. The high blood level of leucine needs to be urgently lowered by haemodialysis. Catabolism must be inhibited and anabolism stimulated by giving high concentrations of i.v. glucose in addition to an infusion of low-dose insulin. Lifelong management includes restriction of natural protein and supplementation with amino acids, vitamins and minerals, and there needs to be regular follow-up in a specialist centre. Leucine, isoleucine and valine (as essential amino acids) need to be included in small amounts in the diet.

Maple syrup urine disease is an autosomal recessive disorder caused by a deficiency of branched chain keto acid dehydrogenase. This results in the accumulation of α-ketoacids (2-oxo-isocaproate, 2-oxo-3methylvaleric acid and 2-oxo-isovalerate) as well as the branched chain amino acids from which they are derived – leucine, isoleucine and valine, respectively. The odour of maple syrup, due to 2-oxo-3-methylvaleric acid, is detected in the urine, sweat and saliva. A urine spot test with 2,4-dinitrophenylhydrazine indicates the presence of ketoacids. The disease is very rare (1 in 185 000). It presents mainly in the newborn period with an acute encephalopathy in the form of lethargy, vomiting, poor feeding, hyper- or hypotonia, fits and coma. A significant metabolic acidosis or hypoglycaemia is not always present. The combination of a progressive encephalopathy with an absence of significant acidosis, hypoglycaemia or hyperammonaemia suggests the diagnosis. There is a marked increase of valine, leucine and isoleucine concentrations in the plasma. Patients with significant encephalopathy require full intensive care. An emergency regimen needs to be devised for parents to use in the event of an intercurrent illness when there is a serious risk of metabolic decompensation.

Patients should be monitored by urine testing with dinitrophenylhydrazine. Urine levels correlate with plasma levels. Mortality from the classic form is up to 20%, death usually being associated with encephalopathic episodes and cerebral oedema. Those surviving an episode often have high morbidity with significant learning difficulties and spastic diplegia.

A 1-year-old boy was referred to the hospital by his GP with a short history of polyuria and 'drinking the bathwater'. His mother also suffered with similar symptoms and received treatment for this. On examination, the child appeared very well apart from a sticky left eye. Initial results showed:

Na 154 mmol/l
K 3.9 mmol/l
Bicarbonate 27 mmol/l
Urea 2.1 mmol/l
Creatinine 25 mmol/l
Glucose 4 mmol/l
Osmolality 309 mOsm/kg
Urine osmolality 283 mOsm/kg

What are the most likely diagnoses?

SELECT *TWO* ANSWERS ONLY

i. Diabetes mellitus
ii. Renal tubular acidosis type 1
iii. Renal tubular acidosis type 2
iv. Hypernatraemic dehydration
v. Water overload
vi. Central diabetes insipidus
vii. Nephrogenic diabetes insipidus
viii. Excess salt ingestion
ix. Bartter syndrome
x. Psychogenic polydipsia

vi. Central diabetes insipidus
vii. Nephrogenic diabetes insipidus

Confirmation (and to distinguish between the two possible diagnoses) is made with a water deprivation test with desmopressin.

Central diabetes insipidus may be inherited as an autosomal dominant or autosomal recessive disease. The boy's presenting symptoms are consistent with diabetes insipidus, diabetes mellitus and psychogenic polydipsia. However, in compulsive water drinking, serum Na (and osmolality) is usually normal or low. Diabetes mellitus in this situation is ruled out by the normal serum glucose. Central and nephrogenic diabetes insipidus can only be distinguished by a water deprivation test followed by desmopressin injection. In the former, the osmolality of urine shows a striking increase after DDAVP, whereas in nephrogenic diabetes insipidus, the urine remains dilute. Central diabetes insipidus is usually an acquired rather than an inherited condition. In our child, the disease followed an autosomal dominant pattern with several members of the mother's family being similarly affected. Occasionally, it may form part of the autosomal recessive Wolfram syndrome (DIDMOAD) when it is associated with diabetes mellitus, optic atrophy and deafness.

Primary nephrogenic diabetes insipidus is usually inherited as an X-linked recessive disease where male infants present with dramatic polyuria and polydipsia. Females with the defect have milder symptoms that may not be detected until later life.

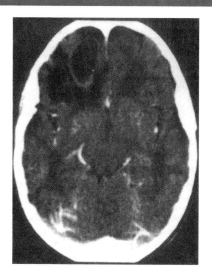

Fig 4.17

A 7-year-old boy was admitted because of increasing lethargy and tiredness over 7 days. Over the last 12 h, he had been refusing food, vomiting and experiencing headache. Three weeks before, he had had a cold, conjunctivitis and otitis media, and that was treated with a course of amoxycillin. Immediately following his admission, he had a generalised seizure lasting 3-4 min. Fundal examination shows bilateral papilloedema. A contrast CT scan of brain is shown.

What is the most likely diagnosis?

SELECT *ONE* ANSWER ONLY

- i. Astrocytoma
- ii. Demyelinating disease
- iii. Brain abscess
- iv. Benign intracranial hypertension
- v. Subacute sclerosing panencephalitis
- vi. Tuberculous meningitis

ANSWER TO CASE 4.17

iii. Brain abscess

The CT scan shows a large low attenuation area over the right frontal cortex, with a thin, enhanced ring shadow. These findings, in conjunction with the history, are most consistent with a diagnosis of a brain abscess.

Management involves urgent transfer to paediatric intensive care unit after stabilising, with urgent neurosurgical referral. He should be treated with i.v. broad-spectrum antibiotics (ceftazidime + flucloxacillin + metronidazole); i.v. dexamethasone will help reduce oedema and anticonvulsants are needed to control and prevent further seizures. Fluids should be used judiciously and electrolytes need close monitoring.

Brain abscess usually presents with headache, vomiting, lethargy, fever and fits. Papilloedema is common and there may be focal neurological signs. Common predisposing factors are otitis media, mastoiditis, sinusitis and underlying cyanotic congenital heart disease, but it may occur without any predisposing factors. The organisms most frequently isolated are microaerophillic streptococci and staphylococcus aureus. Mixed organisms may be involved. Neurosurgical referral is urgently needed for drainage of pus to relieve mass effect and also to identify the organism involved. Pending culture, broad-spectrum i.v. antibiotics should be given and these may have to be continued for several weeks. Neurosurgical intervention depends upon location and stage of abscess, response to antibiotic therapy and clinical condition. Multiple small abscesses require aggressive medical treatment. A single and encapsulated abscess may need total excision. Mortality varies between 11 and 15%. Permanent neurological deficits vary between 45 and 65%.

CASE 4.18

A 3-year-old boy presented to A&E with an 8 h history of pain in his hands and feet, and 1 h of not moving them and not walking. He had been lethargic the previous day, febrile overnight, and vomited once. Three days before, he had returned from 6 weeks in India, where he had had several weeks of diarrhoea. His diet included dairy products, meat and vegetables.

His temperature was 38°C. He was alert with no meningism. His wrists and fingers were flexed. The rest of his examination was normal. His growth parameters were normal. Investigation showed: Hb 9.1 g/dl, WBC 15.6 × 10⁹/l, neutrophils 12.0 × 10⁹/l, platelets 350 × 10⁹/l, CRP 46 mg/l, Na 139 mmol/l, K 4.0 mmol/l, creatinine 50 μmol/l, urea 2.8 mmol/l, Ca (total) 1.58 mmol/l, phosphate 1.53 mmol/l, albumin 40 g/l, Mg 0.18 mmol/l.

What was the cause of his paralysis?

SELECT *ONE* ANSWER ONLY

   i. Guillain–Barre syndrome
  ii. Poliomyelitis
 iii. Tetanus
 iv. Hypomagnesaemia
  v. Hypocalcaemia
 vi. Paratyphoid

ANSWER TO CASE 4.18

iv. Hypomagnesaemia

This boy's tetany is caused by hypomagnesaemia. Second to potassium, magnesium is the most important intracellular cation. Half is in bone and almost all the rest is in the cells of the soft tissues. Less than 1% is in the extracellular fluid. Hypomagnesaemia almost always indicates total body depletion. A child's daily requirement is 0.5–1.0 mmol/kg per 24 h. The usual cause of deficiency is increased intestinal loss (malabsorption or fistulae) with or without a reduced dietary intake. In this patient, the cause was believed to be the prolonged diarrhoea. Occasionally, an increase in urinary excretion (either intrinsic renal tubular disorders or diuretic usage) may result in deficiency. Other causes are cirrhosis and chronic mineralocorticoid excess. The normal range for plasma magnesium in infants is 0.6–0.9 mmol/l, and in older children and adults, 0.75–1.0 mmol/l. Since magnesium is required for both parathyroid hormone secretion and its action on target tissues, magnesium deficiency can cause hypocalcaemia, features of both hypoparathyroidism and pseudohypoparathyroidism, and render patients insensitive to the treatment of hypocalcaemia with vitamin D or calcium. Both hypophosphataemia and hypokalaemia may also be present, but all these abnormalities usually respond to magnesium.

Treatment involves calcium and magnesium replacement; initially i.v., then orally.

CASE 4.19

A 3-week-old infant presents with increasing jaundice, abdominal distension, a 3 cm palpable liver and a palpable spleen tip. She is noted to have several small haemangiomas over her body. Her stools are variably pale and her urine dark. She has mild clinical anaemia with a moderate tachycardia at rest.

Her LFTs are as follows:
Bilirubin 185 μmol/L (Conjugated fraction 94 μmol/L)

ALT 58 U/L	ALP 785 U/L
AST 74 U/L	Albumin 40 g/L
GGT 403 U/L	

What is the most likely diagnosis?

SELECT *ONE* ANSWER ONLY

i. Neuroblastoma
ii. Biliary atresia
iii. Wilson's disease
iv. Gilbert's syndrome
v. Hepatic haemangioma
vi. Neonatal haemachromatosis

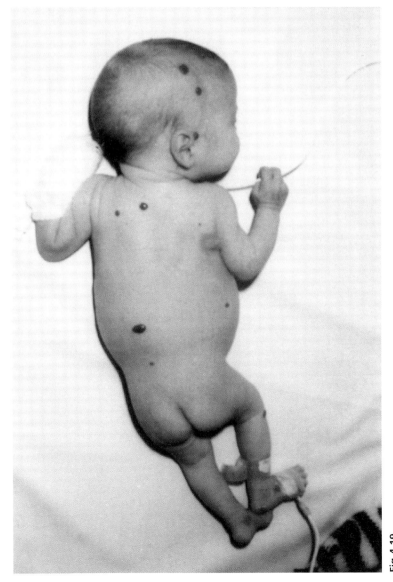

Fig 4.19

ANSWER TO CASE 4.19

v. Hepatic haemangioma.

Fifty per cent of children with hepatic vascular tumours also have cutaneous haemangiomas. Liver haemangioendotheliomas present with the above features, the median age at presentation being 1 month and 70% of infants having high output cardiac failure on presentation. The diagnosis would be supported by the presence on clinical examination of a bruit over the liver. The investigations required usually include liver ultrasound, Doppler imaging, contrast CT and arteriography.

Complications include congestive heart failure, consumptive coagulopathy and microangiopathic anaemia. There may also be increasing mass effects: abdominal distension, obstructive jaundice, vomiting due to GI tract obstruction.

Treatment depends on symptoms. Medical treatment for symptomatic, but non-life-threatening lesions with steroids or α-interferon and for life-threatening lesions, embolisation, hepatic artery ligation or surgical resection.

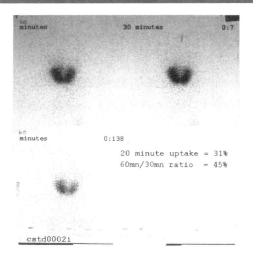

Fig 4.20

A 2-week-old baby boy was referred urgently to the endocrine clinic as he had been found to have a TSH of 70 IU/ml on the neonatal screening test. He was born by normal vaginal delivery at term and is bottle-fed. He is not jaundiced or constipated. There is a family history of deafness with two of his mother's cousins wearing hearing aids from early childhood. The older sibling of the patient has diabetes. The mother's grandmother was thought to have a swelling in her neck.

On examination, the baby was found to have a large swelling in his neck. The rest of his systemic examination was normal.

The figure shown is of a perchlorate discharge scan showing rapid uptake of radioactive iodine with 45% discharge of iodine 1 h after perchlorate was given.

What is the diagnosis?

SELECT *ONE* ANSWER ONLY
   i. Congenital hypothyroidism secondary to thyroid agenesis
   ii. Congenital hypothyroidism secondary to iodine deficiency
   iii. Congenital hypothyroidism secondary to dyshormonogenesis
   iv. Normal perchlorate scan

ANSWER TO CASE 4.20

iii. Congenital hypothyroidism secondary to dyshormonogenesis

In the UK, goitre is a rare finding in the neonatal period, which suggests an inborn error in thyroid hormone synthesis (iodine deficiency occurs in some areas and can also present with goitre). These defects are commoner in consanguineous marriages. The perchlorate discharge scan is a useful tool for detection of dyshormonogenesis. The perchlorate ion competes with iodide for trapping by the thyroid follicular cell plasma membrane and the discharge of iodine occurs, which can be monitored by release of radiation from the gland. Further investigations include FT4 and repeat TSH, ultrasound scan of the thyroid gland, a radio-iodine scan and a hearing test.

Congenital hypothyroidism is inadequate thyroid hormone production in newborn infants. This can occur because of an anatomic defect in the gland, an inborn error of thyroid metabolism, or iodine deficiency. The incidence is 1:3-4000. The thyroid gland uses tyrosine and iodine to make thyroxine (T4) and triiodothyronine (T3). Iodide is actively taken into the thyroid follicular cells and then oxidized to iodine by thyroid peroxidase. Organification occurs when iodine is attached to tyrosine molecules attached to thyroglobulin, finally forming tetraiodothyronine (i.e. T4). TSH activates enzymes needed to cleave T3 and T4 from thyroglobulin.

Inborn errors of thyroid metabolism can result in congenital hypothyroidism in children with anatomically normal thyroid glands. Iodine deficiency during fetal and postnatal life causes goitre and hypothyroidism.

Aetiologies: excluding iodine deficiency, congenital hypothyroidism can caused by:
- Dysgenesis of the thyroid gland
  - Agenesis of or ectopic thyroid
- Inborn errors of thyroid hormone metabolism (dyshormonogenesis)
  - TSH receptor abnormalities, abnormal iodide uptake, peroxidase or organification defects (i.e. inability to convert iodine to iodide) such as Pendred sydrome – associated with congenital deafness
- Thyroid hormone resistance (thyroid hormone receptor abnormalities)
- Maternal autoimmune disease (transient or permanent)
- TSH or TRH deficiencies, e.g. hypopituitarism
- Iatrogenic causes (maternal use of thioamides, iodine excess, radioactive iodine therapy)

Chapter

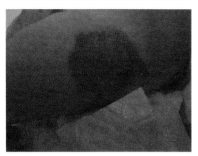

Fig 5.1.A

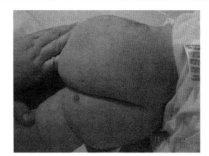

Fig 5.1.B

A distraught single mother brought her 8 month old to the A&E department very worried about lesions that looked like burns and just appeared out of nowhere (Fig. 5.1.A). The child was fully immunised, born to non-consanguineous parents and bottle-fed. The child was not left unsupervised at all according to the mother, and she clearly recalls the absence of these lesions 24 h before.

While an inpatient, newer lesions appeared (Fig. 5.1.B).

Which of the following should be considered in the differential diagnosis?

SELECT *TWO* ANSWERS ONLY

   i. Scarlet fever
  ii. Pomphylox
 iii. Impetigo
  iv. Incontinentia pigmenti
   v. Dystrophic epidermolysis bullosa
  vi. Staphylococcal scalded skin syndrome
 vii. Bullous pemphigoid

ANSWERS TO CASE 5.1

  iii. Impetigo
  vi. Staphylococcal scalded skin syndrome

Differential diagnosis of generalised exfoliation includes drug-induced and virus-mediated toxic epidermal necrolysis, burns, epidermolysis bullosa, bullous erythema multiforme and diffuse cutaneous mastocytosis as well as staphylococcal scalded skin syndrome (SSSS) and impetigo.

Treatment of SSSS involves i.v. flucloxacillin and supportive therapy. SSSS is a disease primarily affecting infants and young children. In the infant, the lesions are mostly found on the perineum or periumbilically, or both, while the extremities are more commonly affected in older children. The disease begins with erythema and fever, followed by formation of large fluid-filled bullae, which quickly rupture on slightest pressure (Nikolsky sign) to leave extensive areas of denuded skin. The form and severity of SSSS will vary with the route of delivery of the toxin to the skin, ranging from the localised bullous impetigo to generalised SSSS involving the entire skin surface. In the latter, patients are prone to poor temperature control, extensive fluid losses and secondary infections. They may also develop sepsis and present with hypotension, neutropenia and respiratory distress. Antibiotic treatment with β-lactamase-resistant semisynthetic penicillins such as flucloxacillin is usually effective.

CASE 5.2

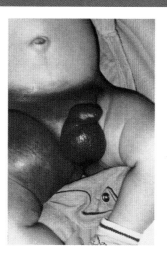

Fig 5.1

A 3-week-old baby presented with a large bruise-like swelling overlying the right thigh that had developed quickly over 3 days. The baby had been delivered by Caesarean section for failure to progress. At birth, a small mark had been noted at the same site. It was thought to be due to trauma during the Caesarean section. The baby was given intramuscular vitamin K in the contralateral thigh. On examination, the leg was held in flexion and there was a large hard mass that appeared to involve the upper thigh, lower abdominal wall and scrotum.

The child appeared otherwise well with no circulatory compromise.

The results of investigations were:
    Hb 7.6 g/dl
    Platelets 22 × 10⁹/l ↓
    WCC 12.4 × 10⁹/l

The blood film was reported as showing red cell fragmentation and no evidence of platelet clumping.
Clotting profile:
    APTT >180 s
    PT >30 s
    Fibrinogen >0.1 g/l

What is the most likely diagnosis?

SELECT *ONE* ANSWER ONLY
   i. Spreading cellulitis
  ii. Maternal thrombocytopaenia with transplacental transfer of antibodies
 iii. Von Willebrand's syndrome
  iv. Kasabach-Merritt syndrome
   v. Haemophilia B

ANSWERS CASE 5.2

iv. Kasabach–Merritt syndrome

This child has apparently developed a large swelling, which may be a haematoma so clotting investigations are mandatory. FBC will help to show whether a significant amount of blood has been lost. Ultrasound of the lesion will help to quantify its size and extent – in this child, it extended up to the lower poles of both kidneys in the retroperitoneum.

Later MRI enhanced with contrast will be helpful in the management of this condition.

The diagnosis here is Kasabach–Merritt syndrome. This child has a rapidly proliferating haemangioma (histology when performed showed this to be kaposiform haemangioendothelioma) and a consumptive coagulopathy.

Management options include high-dose oral steroids. Only correct clotting abnormalities and platelet count if the child is actively bleeding. If the lesion does not respond to oral steroids then i.v. methylprednisolone may be required. Other possible therapies include vincristine, α-interferon, radiotherapy, amputation and embolisation.

The prognosis of these lesions is very variable. Some authors quote 20-30% mortality. Older papers quote 60%. It is probably dependent on the initial size of the lesion with retroperitoneal lesions faring worse.

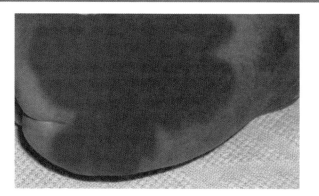

Fig 5.3

A newborn baby presented at birth with the skin lesion shown.

a. What is the principal lesion?
   SELECT *ONE* ANSWER ONLY
   i. Port-wine stain (naevus flammeus)
   ii. Telangectatic naevus
   iii. Giant melanocytic naevus
   iv. Mongolian blue spot
   v. Strawberry naevus

b. Which two investigations would you request?
   SELECT *TWO* ANSWERS ONLY
   i. Karyotype
   ii. Head MRI
   iii. Spinal MRI
   iv. FBC
   v. Head ultrasound
   vi. Lumbar X-ray

ANSWERS TO CASE 5.3

a. i. Port-wine stain (naevus flammeus)
b. iii. Spinal MRI
    iv. FBC

This photograph shows a port-wine stain of the lumbosacral area. Port-wine stains are present at birth. They are large, irregular, deep red macular lesions and represent a vascular malformation involving mature dilated dermal capillaries. The lesions are sharply circumscribed and vary tremendously in size. Most of the lesions are present on the head and neck, most are unilateral, and in general the lesions deepen in colour with age. The most effective treatment is pulsed dye laser therapy, which avoids thermal injury to the surrounding tissue and leads to improvement without scarring. Major morbidities (in the absence of syndromic or other associations) include poor self-image and traumatic bleeding.

Investigations required include an MRI of the lumbosacral spine (maybe ultrasound of the lumbosacral area) and a FBC to exclude Kasabach–Merritt syndrome (haemangioma associated with thrombocytopenia).

Haemangiomas over the lumbosacral area are associated with spinal dysraphism, which is a general term for coexistent vertebral and spinal cord defects. Spina bifida occulta is the most common and benign defect, but other lesions include intradural and extra-dural lipomas, cysts, teratomas and tethering of the spinal cord. MRI of the spine is the investigation of choice.

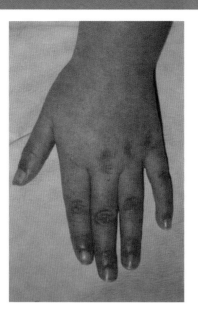

Fig 5.4

It is the middle of a particularly hot summer when a 5-year-old girl presents with a 2-month history of being profoundly miserable and tired. Her parents have noticed a rash on her face but felt this was due to sun exposure. Previously a very active child, she is now lethargic, and her mother has noticed particular problems on getting out of bed and going upstairs. Her GP has taken some routine blood samples and was surprised to find that her CRP level was 156. The rash found on her hands is shown. Neurologically, she has profound proximal muscle weakness.

What is the most likely diagnosis?

SELECT *ONE* ANSWER ONLY

   i. Juvenile dermatomyositis
  ii. Myotonic dystrophy
 iii. Post-viral syndrome
 iv. Guillain–Barre syndrome
  v. Systemic lupus erythematosus
 vi. Polymyalgia rheumatica

ANSWER TO CASE 5.4

i. Juvenile dermatomyositis.

Juvenile dermatomyositis is a multisystem disorder that results in inflammation of the skin, striated muscle and gastrointestinal tract. The exact aetiology is unknown, but research is focused on abnormalities of cell-mediated immunity and immune complex disease; infection may also have a role. The onset is common between the ages of 4 and 10 years, and the condition is more frequent in girls.

Juvenile dermatomyositis usually presents with a combination of malaise, fatigue, fever, profound flexor muscle weakness and rash. The rash is often pathognomic, with a heliotrope discolouration around the eyes, Gottren's papules (shiny, erythematous plaques on the extensor surfaces of the finger joints and other extensor surfaces) and nailfold capillary loop dilatation. The flexor muscle weakness is shown by a positive Gower's sign, an inability to flex the neck off pillows, difficulty going upstairs, etc. One of the complications of this disease is calcinosis (subcutaneous or within the muscle layers). Dermatomyositis can also be complicated by dysphagia, pulmonary restriction, muscle atrophy and contractures and lipoatrophy.

Laboratory tests often (although not always) show a high level of muscle enzymes (creatinine kinase) as well as elevated inflammatory markers. An electromyogram can also be helpful. Magnetic resonance mapping shows myositis. If the diagnosis is uncertain, an ultrasound-guided muscle biopsy can be performed.

Treatment must be multidisciplinary. Medical treatment aims to reduce inflammation using prednisolone, hydroxychloroquine, methotrexate (and other second-line agents) and immunoglobulin. The outcome varies according to the course of the disease. Many have limited disease and the outcome is excellent; a small percentage, however, develop aggressive disease and require ongoing support. Mortality is approximately 5% and usually follows pulmonary insufficiency, acute gastrointestinal bleeding or sepsis.

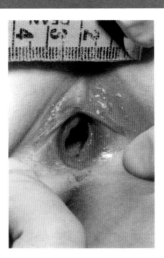

Fig 5.5

A 5-year-old girl was brought to the paediatrician by her professional parents. Her symptoms included intermittent dribbling, dysuria and urgency. Her GP had treated her with several courses of antibiotics for symptoms suggestive of urinary tract infections. Only one of numerous mid-stream urine specimens had isolated organisms. Her school work was deteriorating. Her growth and blood pressure were normal. Inspection of the urogenital region revealed no dribbling and looked as shown.

What abnormal features can you see?

SELECT *TWO* ANSWERS ONLY

  i. Gaping and scarred hymen
 ii. Threadworms
iii. Lichen sclerosis
 iv. Posterior healed transection of hymen
  v. Foreign body

ANSWERS TO CASE 5.5

i. Gaping and scarred hymen
iv. Posterior healed transection of hymen

The photograph shows a markedly attenuated scarred hymen with a posterior healed transection at the 7 o'clock position. There is also a gaping hymenal orifice.

These findings are consistent with penetrative trauma and probable sexual abuse.

Further steps to be taken include:
- a full paediatric assessment for evidence of associated physical abuse
- explanation of concerns to parents and why child protection services must be contacted
- referral to a paediatrician experienced in dealing with sexual abuse
- screening for sexually transmitted disease
- evaluation of siblings should be considered
- involvement of the child and family mental health team

Child sexual abuse in young children can present with symptoms suggestive of urinary tract infection, urinary incontinence, deterioration in school work and behavioural changes. Allegations by young children of intrafamilial sexual abuse are uncommon.

The attenuated hymen which indicates loss of tissue and the posterior healed transection are clinical evidence of penetrative trauma. A gaping hymenal orifice should not be used as a sole basis for diagnosis as assessment is not always reliable. The findings in this child are not possible to date.

Although the parents have to be informed about suspicion, utmost care should be taken to ensure that the child is not put at further risk. The child's welfare is paramount and screening for sexually transmitted disease should be carried out. A police surgeon may be asked to assist a paediatrician who doesn't have relevant forensic expertise. As there is no allegation and no clinical evidence of recent assault, forensic samples may not be indicated.

Other siblings may need to be evaluated as it is likely that they may also be being abused. A referral to the mental health team should help with assessing any psychological and emotional needs of the child and family.

CASE 5.6

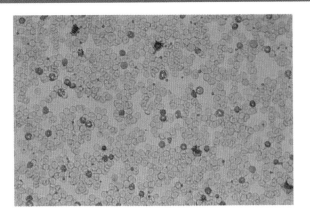

Fig 5.6

A baby was delivered by emergency Caesarean section at 34 weeks' gestation following decreased fetal movements for 2 days and a poorly reactive cardiotocogram. She required full resuscitation and was found to have a Hb of 2.3 g/dl. She was not hydropic and did not have hepatosplenomegaly.

What does this blood film (Kleihauer test) show?

SELECT *ONE* ANSWER ONLY

   i. Acute haemolysis
  ii. Positive Coombs' test
 iii. Microcytic hypochromic anaemia
  iv. Sickling
   v. Feto-maternal haemorrhage
  vi. Haemolytic disease of the newborn

ANSWER TO CASE 5.6

v. Feto-maternal haemorrhage

Profound fetal anaemia can be due to haemorrhage or haemolysis or failure of production, e.g. parvovirus infection. Haemorrhagic causes include fetomaternal transfusions, twin-to-twin transfusions, fetoplacental transfusion at birth, fetal haemorrhage due to placenta praevia, placental abruption or placental injury during Caesarean section. Perinatal haemorrhages can be intracranial, subaponeurotic, intra-abdominal or due to umbilical cord rupture. Absence of hepatosplenomegaly and hydrops makes haemolysis and failure of production unlikely in this case.

Investigations include FBC and film, blood group (maternal and fetal), direct Coombs' test, serum bilirubin, maternal Kleihauer, coagulation screen and ultrasound scans to search for concealed haemorrhage.

The figure shows the Kleihauer test, prepared from the maternal blood film, which has been stained with eosin and treated with acid. The acid elutes adult haemoglobin leaving "ghost cells". Fetal cells retain the stain since fetal haemoglobin is acid resistant. The volume of transfusion can be estimated from a differential count of maternal and fetal cells. This together with a negative direct Coombs' test and normal bilirubin suggest a feto-maternal haemorrhage. In this case, it was an estimated 380 ml. This is greater than the circulating volume of the baby as the fetal red cells may survive many weeks.

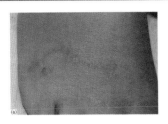 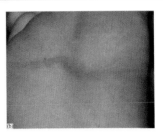

Fig 5.7

A 5-year-old girl returned from a holiday in Jamaica with her parents 4 weeks ago. Her mother reported that an ant had bitten her on the beach. Two weeks later she developed a lesion on her foot. It was itchy and spreading.

a. What is the diagnosis?
   SELECT *ONE* ANSWER ONLY
   i. Schistosomiasis
   ii. Scabies
   iii. Erythema marginatum
   iv. Cutaneous larva migrans
   v. Lyme disease

b. What is the underlying cause?
   SELECT *ONE* ANSWER ONLY
   i. Sarcoptes scabiei
   ii. Streptococcal infection
   iii. Trichuris tricuria
   iv. Borrelia burgdorferi
   v. Ancylostoma braziliense

ANSWERS TO CASE 5.7

a. iv. Cutaneous larva migrans
b. v. Ancylostoma braziliense

This is an example of cutaneous larva migrans. This is caused by skin infestation with hookworm or roundworm larva. Cutaneous larva migrans may well be seen in children in the UK because of increased travel to exotic destinations. The usual agent is *Ancylostoma braziliense*, a hookworm found in cats and dogs. It is endemic in southern areas of the United States, in Central and South America, and in other subtropical areas. *Ancylostoma caninum* is much less common in these areas but is ubiquitous in dogs and cats in Australia. In warm, moist sandy soil the eggs mature into filariform larvae, which penetrate the skin. After a few days the larvae begin migration in the base of the epidermis, moving as much as several centimetres daily. The larva is 1-2 cm beyond the advancing edge of the lesion. Treatment is with thiabendazole. Topical thiabendazole cream is probably the treatment of choice. Oral thiabendazole is associated with gastrointestinal side effects.

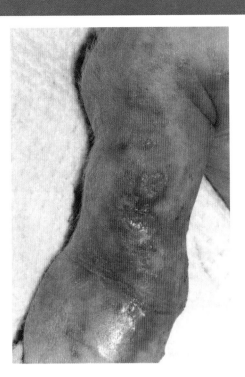

Fig 5.8

A well, term baby girl was reviewed following delivery because of a generalised rash (see photo). Her mother had a history of recurrent miscarriages but this pregnancy had been uncomplicated.

What is the most likely diagnosis?

SELECT *ONE* ANSWER ONLY

   i. Incontinentia pigmenti
  ii. Disseminated herpes simplex infection
 iii. Neonatal urticaria
 iv. Infantile pomphylox
  v. Eczema herpeticum

ANSWER TO CASE 5.8

i. Incontinentia pigmenti

Differential diagnosis of this generalized bullous eruption includes infectious causes, e.g. staphylococcal bullous impetigo, herpes simplex (neonates likely to be unwell), and non-infectious diseases, e.g. incontinentia pigmenti (the diagnosis in this case) and epidermolysis bullosa.

Incontinentia pigmenti, also known as Bloch–Sulzberger syndrome, is a rare disorder characterised by abnormalities in ectodermal tissues including skin, eyes, CNS and dentition. It is inherited as an X-linked dominant disorder which is usually lethal in male fetuses. In the neonatal period, the skin lesions are characteristically bullous and it is an important differential diagnosis in any baby with a vesicular rash.

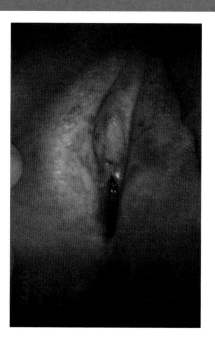

Fig 5.9

A 6-year-old girl was brought to A&E by her mother one evening, who had noted drops of blood on her knickers and "itching below". There was some dysuria, but no discharge. As usual, her uncle had taken her to school that morning. He had reported to her mother that the child had tripped and fallen on a concrete step. The duty paediatric registrar is asked to see her. The figure shows the appearance of her external genitalia.

a. What does the picture show?
   SELECT *ONE* ANSWER ONLY
   i. Vulvitis
   ii. Candida infection
   iii. Cliteromegaly
   iv. (Vulval) lichen sclerosus et atrophicus
   v. Ragged, torn hymen

b. Which important diagnosis must also be considered?
   SELECT *ONE* ANSWER ONLY
   i. Urinary tract infection
   ii. Threadworms
   iii. Sexual abuse
   iv. Trauma
   v. Ovarian failure

a. iv. Lichen sclerosus et atrophicus
b. iii. Sexual abuse

This picture shows haemorrhagic vulval lichen sclerosus et atrophicus. This condition is seen in pre-pubertal girls and post-menopausal women. Initially white papules appear which then join to form plaques. Haemorrhagic areas may also be present. These are part of the disorder and not secondary to scratching. Marked itching and vulval soreness are presenting symptoms, and scratching and rubbing may lead to bleeding of the fragile skin. There may well be a family history of lichen sclerosus. Treatment is with topical steroids. Resolution occurs at or just after the menarche.

The possibility of sexual abuse must also be considered, and in fact, the two conditions may co-exist, as the trauma related to sexual abuse may act as a trigger to developing lichen sclerosus, related to Koebnerization, which is known to occur in this disease. It is important to elicit a full history regarding the extent of the trauma – was it a straddle injury? Did she appear to have painful external genitalia following the incident? Minimal trauma can cause bleeding and acute inflammation in the presence of lichen sclerosus but a straddle injury could explain inflammation or injury to the hymen.

Are there any long-standing concerns about this child from mother or school? For example, any deterioration in schoolwork or behavioural problems. Ask about the dysuria and symptoms of a urinary tract infection, and find out more about the itching – over labia or anus? Night or day, or both? Intermittent or longstanding? Threadworms need to be excluded as a co-existing cause for the itchiness.

General examination, and examination of the external genitalia and anus using a magnifying light source is important; this should be done with the consultant present in child sexual abuse, to avoid repeated examinations. Investigations should include midstream urine to exclude a urinary tract infection, and a tape slide to exclude threadworms. If there is a history of vaginal discharge, a swab should be taken.

The child should be discharged to a place of safety, with careful follow-up. Do bear in mind that it is possible to have a hymen of normal appearance with sexual abuse, and lichen sclerosus and sexual abuse are not mutually exclusive diagnoses.

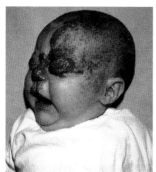

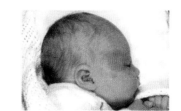

Fig 5.10.2

Fig 5.10.1

a + ii
- Strawberry nevus
- Kass. Merrit

c + i
- port-wine stain
- calcycati of legions

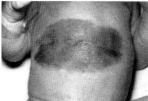

Fig 5.10.3

B + iii
- melanocytic nevus
- premalignant

Choose the name and recognised association of each of these three dermatalogical lesions:

a. Strawberry naevus
b. Melanocytic naevus
c. Port-wine stain

i. May be associated with calcification of the leptomeninges
ii. May be associated with Kasabach–Merritt syndrome
iii. Is potentially premalignant

a = ii
b = iii
c = i

Questions and Answers for the New Format Exam

Figure 5.10.1: **a.** and ii. "Strawberry naevus" and "May be associated with the Kasabach-Merritt syndrome"

Figure 5.10.2: **c.** and i. "Port-wine stain" and "May be associated with calcification of the leptomeninges"

Figure 5.10.3: **b.** and iii. "Melanocytic naevus" and "Is potentially premalignant"

Figure 5.10.1 is a strawberry naevus, the most common of the capillary haemangiomas. It usually presents as a small red papule which develops at or soon after birth, and increases in size for a few years. It then gradually involutes to leave an excellent cosmetic result. The incidence is 1 : 20 babies. A minority will cause problems such as bleeding, ulceration and disfigurement. Other complications are visual impairment or airway obstruction depending on the site of the haemangioma. Rarely the lesion may be extensive and the abnormal vessels may sequester platelets causing thrombocytopaenia and a petechial rash (Kasabach–Merritt syndrome). For lesions likely to cause problems, early treatment with oral or intralesional steroids, α-interferon and laser therapy should be considered.

Figure 5.10.2 is a port-wine stain, a vascular malformation. This has an incidence of 3 : 1000 births. It is a macular red or purple area which often affects one side of the face. It is usually present at birth and stays the same size relative to the head size as the child grows. The condition persists throughout life, becoming darker and thicker with age, and can be very disfiguring. Pulse dye laser therapy is the treatment of choice and younger children respond better. A facial port-wine stain can be associated with angiomatosis and calcification of the leptomeninges over the cerebral cortex. The patient may present with convulsions, hemiplegia and mental retardation (Sturge–Weber syndrome). All children with a facial port-wine stain on the upper part of the face and scalp should have a baseline MRI scan looking for central nervous system involvement.

Figure 5.10.3 is a melanocytic naevus. This naevus is due to a developmental defect causing benign localised proliferation of the melanocytes in the dermis. Melanocytic naevi vary considerably in size and appearance. They are potentially premalignant. Extensive, deeply pigmented, hairy naevi which are present at birth seem more likely to become malignant.

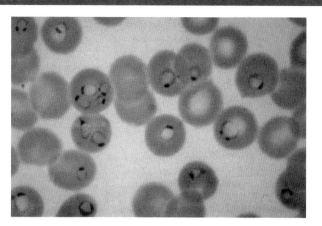

Fig 5.11

A 5-year-old child of Indian parents has recently returned from visiting family in rural India. He has had a fever for 48 h, but has no focal symptoms. On examination he has a temperature of 41°C, with 3 cm splenomegaly, and no rash. He does not appear particularly unwell. Investigations show:

Hb 9.3 g/dl
WBC 10.5 × 10⁹/l
Platelets 200 × 10⁹/l
CRP 8 mg/l

A blood film demonstrating the condition is shown.

What is the diagnosis?

SELECT *ONE* ANSWER ONLY

  i. Typhoid fever
 ii. Paratyphoid
iii. P. falciparum malaria .
 iv. P. vivax malaria
  v. Dengue fever
 vi. Yellow fever

ANSWER TO CASE 5.11

iii. P. falciparum malaria

Important information to elicit to aid in making the diagnosis would be any history of antimalarial prophylaxis, which antimalarials had been used, and if so whether they were taken at least a week prior to travelling and 4 weeks following return. Also, any contact with known febrile illness may also be relevant.

Investigations should include FBC, differential, and thick and thin blood films for malaria parasites which need to be done rapidly, as complications may occur within hours of symptoms first occurring. As a negative film does not exclude malaria, at least three films should be taken in potential cases. Alternative differential diagnoses (e.g. typhoid fever) may prompt other investigations, particularly culture of blood and urine. Rapid blood antigen detection methods for malaria are now available, and are becoming a useful adjunct to aid diagnosis. The diagnosis here is P. falciparum malaria, as there are multiple ring forms in red cells on the thin film.

Managing the child with malaria needs to be undertaken in hospital. Although chloroquine was historically the drug of choice for uncomplicated malaria, it is no longer recommended as resistance is common worldwide. Quinine for 5 days or until the blood film is negative, followed by a single dose of sulphadoxine pyremethamine (Fansidar) is the appropriate treatment for imported malaria managed in the UK, and in an uncomplicated case could be given orally in hospital. An alternative treatment for children over 2 years would be mefloquine. Up to date, telephone advice on the management of malaria, (and its prophylaxis) is available from the Schools of Tropical Medicine in Liverpool and London.

There are about 300 cases of malaria in children each year in the UK, half of whom did not take antimalarial prophylaxis. However, chemo-prophylaxis does not guarantee protection against malaria. With increasing antimalarial resistance, breakthrough infection is well recognised. Antimalarials should be continued for 4 weeks after returning from a malarious area. For this child with P. falciparum malaria no further treatment is required, but a film should be examined at the end of treatment, and after 4 weeks (or with subsequent fever) to ensure eradication. Had the child developed P. vivax infection, this is mostly chloroquine sensitive, but resistant strains are described from India. P. vivax also requires a 2-3 week course of primaquine orally to clear the hypnozoite stage from the liver. Dormant hypnozoites of P. vivax cause relapse, but are not present in the life cycle of P. falciparum. This child could have a mixed infection with P. vivax, which may declare itself some months later after treatment has stopped.

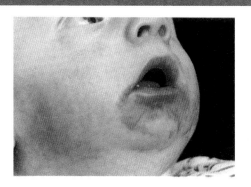

Fig 5.12

This 6-month-old male infant was referred to a paediatric outpatient clinic for eczema in the perioral, post auricular and perineal regions. He also had intermittent diarrhoea. The use of various moisturisers and topical hydrocortisone cream did not improve it. He had fallen below the 2nd centile for weight and was on the 10th centile for length. On examination, he had scanty scalp hair.

a. What is the rash due to?
   SELECT *ONE* ANSWER ONLY
   i. Seborrhoeic eczema
   ii. Iron deficiency
   iii. Zinc deficiency
   iv. Latex allergy from teat of bottle
   v. Infected eczema
   vi. Staphylococcal infection

b. What are the other manifestations of this condition?
   SELECT *TWO* ANSWERS ONLY
   i. Constipation
   ii. Nail pitting
   iii. Corneal opacities
   iv. Irritability
   v. Anorexia and failure to thrive
   vi. Deranged coagulation

c. How may the condition be inherited?
   SELECT *ONE* ANSWER ONLY
   i. Autosomal recessive
   ii. No genetic link
   iii. Autosomal dominant
   iv. X-linked acquired form

ANSWERS TO CASE 5.12

a. iii. Zinc deficiency
b. iv. Irritability
   v. Anorexia and failure to thrive
c.   i. Autosomal recessive inheritance

Zinc deficiency can be either congenital or acquired. The acquired form of zinc deficiency is more common. The rash due to zinc deficiency has a peculiar perioral distribution that is smooth and shiny unlike the rash of eczema, which usually occurs in the flexures in this age group. This infant's zinc level was 2 μmol (normal range 8–16 μmol).

Other manifestations of zinc deficiency include acrodermatitis, alopecia, diarrhoea, poor wound healing, neurological disturbances like irritability or lethargy, impaired cell-mediated immunity and chemotaxis with recurrent infection, anorexia and failure to thrive, hypogonadism and corneal changes and nyctalopia (impaired vision in the dark).

Zinc deficiency can be acquired secondary to nutritional deficiency, but can also be inherited as a congenital form called acrodermatitis enteropathica. It results from an as yet uncertain defect in the intestinal absorption of zinc, and is inherited in an autosomal recessive manner.

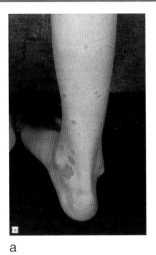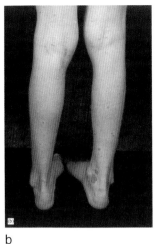

a   b

Fig 5.13

An 8-year-old girl was admitted with a 2-day history of intermittent crampy abdominal pain and passing fresh bloody stools. Other than seasonal colds she had been well, with no recent weight loss, no other bleeding sites and no previous episodes. Initial investigations revealed normal FBC and film, normal serum U&E, albumin 32 g/l and other LFTs were normal.

a. Which of the following would be included in your initial differential diagnosis?
SELECT THE *THREE* BEST ANSWERS
  i. Acute appendicitis
  ii. Giardiasis infection
  iii. Salmonella infection
  iv. Meckel's diverticulum
  v. Intussusception
  vi. Inflammatory bowel disease
  vii. Diverticular disease

b. What other investigations would you do initially?
SELECT *THREE* ANSWERS ONLY
  i. Coagulation screen
  ii. Abdominal X-ray
  iii. Upper GI endoscopy
  iv. Inflammatory markers
  v. Colonoscopy
  vi. Abdominal ultrasound scan
  vii. Stool for faecal occult blood

Her symptoms settled spontaneously and she was discharged after 48 h to be seen again as an out-patient. However, 2 days later she presented with a rash as shown in Figure 5.13.a and b.

c. What is the most likely diagnosis?
SELECT *ONE* ANSWER ONLY
  i. Inflammatory bowel disease
  ii. Polyarteritis
  iii. Henoch–Schönlein Purpura
  iv. Von Willebrand's disease
  v. Haemophilia A

ANSWERS TO CASE 5.13

a. iii. Salmonella infection
   iv. Meckel's diverticulum
   v. Intussusception
b. i. Coagulation screen
   iv. Inflammatory markers
   vi. Abdominal ultrasound scan
c. iii. Henoch–Schönlein Purpura

Causes which need to be considered in this case include infective (salmonella, E. coli, etc.), surgical (fissure, polyp, intussusception, Meckel's diverticulum) and inflammatory bowel disease.

Stool should be sent for microscopy and culture plus virology. If bleeding is significant a sample should be sent for cross-match.

Inflammatory markers (as well as routine FBC, U&E, LFTs and coagulation) should also be checked.

An ultrasound scan is generally of more help than an X-ray (which also confers a dose of radiation).

The rash, which is a non-tender purpuric rash (mainly on extensor aspects of legs and buttocks) is Henoch–Schonlein Purpura. It is important to measure blood pressure and dip the urine for blood and protein, both of which signal renal involvement, which will need follow-up.

GI involvement is common in Henoch–Schönlein Purpura, and bleeding from the gut may be occult or frank, secondary to the vasculitic process or to intussusception of the colon. The colicky abdominal pain may be treated with simple analgesia and some elect to treat with steroids if the symptoms are severe. The associated complication of intussusception can be difficult to rule out and if in doubt paediatric radiological and surgical opinions should be sought.

The prognosis for gut involvement is good, with resolution of the symptoms over weeks to months as the vasculitic process settles.

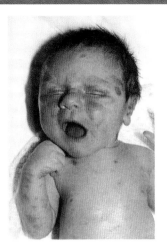

Fig 5.14

A term baby boy delivered by SVD was noted on routine post-natal examination to have an unusual rash. His mother was a 22-year-old primigravida with no significant past medical or family history. This pregnancy had been uncomplicated.

a. What further investigations should be requested on the mother?
   SELECT *TWO* ANSWERS ONLY
   i. Anti-Ro antibodies
   ii. Rheumatoid factor
   iii. Antinuclear antibodies
   iv. Anti-La antibodies
   v. Viral titres
   vi. ECG

b. What further investigations should be requested on the baby?
   SELECT *TWO* ANSWERS ONLY
   i. FBC
   ii. Blood cultures
   iii. EEG
   iv. CXR
   v. ECG
   vi. Cranial ultrasound scan

ANSWERS TO CASE 5.14

a. i. Anti-Ro antibodies
    iv. Anti-La antibodies
b. i. FBC
    v. ECG

The abnormalities shown are a butterfly facial rash and discoid erythematous patches.

Differential diagnosis includes neonatal SLE or staphylococcal skin sepsis. To investigate for maternal SLE, anti-Ro and anti-La antibodies must be checked.

Neonatal investigations include an ECG for evidence of heart block, FBC for evidence of thrombocytopenia, and LFTs for evidence of hepatitis.

Neonatal SLE can present in infants of asymptomatic mothers (as in this case) as well as in those with established disease. It occurs as a result of transplacental transfer of maternal autoantibodies, particularly Ro and La autoantibodies. It is characterised by one or more of: congenital heart block, cardiomyopathy, cutaneous lesions, hepatobiliary disease and thrombocytopenia.

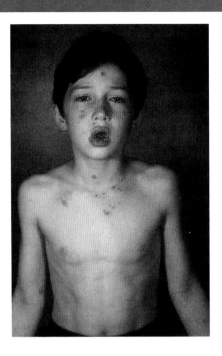

Fig 5.15

This 8-year-old boy presented with a widespread rash following a mild upper respiratory tract infection, associated with conjunctivitis and oral lesions.

a. What is the most likely diagnosis?
   SELECT *ONE* ANSWER ONLY
   i. Toxic epidermal necrolysis
   ii. Stevens–Johnson syndrome •
   iii. Gingivostomatitis
   iv. Herpes zoster
   v. Reiter disease

b. Choose two known causes of this rash:
   SELECT *TWO* ANSWERS ONLY
   i. Vancomycin
   ii. Latex allergy
   iii. Gluten enteropathy
   iv. Leukaemia ›
   v. Streptococcal infection •
   vi. Varicella infection

ANSWERS TO CASE 5.15

a. ii. Stevens–Johnson syndrome
b. iv. Leukaemia
    v. Streptococcal infection

This child has Stevens–Johnson syndrome (erythema multiforme major). It is generally regarded as a hypersensitivity reaction to various medications, infections and toxic substances, such as nitrobenzene, and radiation therapy. Drugs implicated in its aetiology include penicillin, sulphonamides, isoniazid, tetracyclines, phenytoin, carbamazepine, captopril, aspirin and etoposide. Infections include herpes simplex 1 and 2, mycoplasma pneumonia, group B strep, BCG vaccine, yersinia and enteroviruses. It is also seen in patients with leukaemia and lymphoma. Stevens–Johnson syndrome is a serious disorder in which at least two mucous membranes, as well as skin, are involved. Clinically it presents as a widespread erythematous rash with target lesions (central vesicular or erythematous area surrounded by concentric rings of pallor and erythema), purulent conjunctivitis and lesions on the oral mucosa. The classic lesions usually appear following a prodromal respiratory illness. New lesions occur over 1-4 weeks with healing over 6 weeks. Treatment might include i.v. fluids, systemic and topical antibiotics and skin care.

Differential diagnosis of this rash would include toxic epidermal necrolysis, gingivostomatitis, Reiter disease and benign mucous membrane pemphigoid.

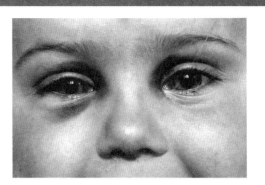

Fig 5.16

This 2-year-old presented to the A&E department with bilateral conjunctival haemorrhages, and periorbital bruises. She attended with her mother and stepfather who said they first noticed her appearance when she woke up in the morning. There was no history of trauma. The parents reported that she was happy and well in herself, except for a nagging harsh cough for the previous 2 weeks. Apart from the appearance of her eyes, her examination was entirely normal. A blood count showed:

Hb 10.0 g/dl
WCC 25 × 10⁹/l
Neutrophils 3.1 × 10⁹/l
Lymphocytes 21.2 × 10⁹/l
Platelets 227 × 10⁹/l

What other investigation would you perform?

SELECT *ONE* ANSWER ONLY

i. Blood culture
ii. Pernasal swab
iii. Urine for catecholamines
iv. Skull X-ray
v. Nasopharyngeal aspirate

ANSWER TO CASE 5.16

ii. Pernasal swab

This little girl had pertussis infection (whooping cough). A pernasal swab should be sent for Bordetella pertussis.

The possibility of non-accidental injury must be excluded. However, examination was otherwise entirely normal and there were no other concerns. Should there be any concerns, a skeletal survey and ophthalmological examination should be arranged, and referral made to social services. On observation, her cough was paroxysmal in nature, with occasional, but definite episodes of whooping. The lymphocytosis further supported the diagnosis, and after 7 days, her pernasal swab confirmed growth of *Bordetella pertussis*. Conjunctival haemorrhages are a recognised complication of whooping cough, and used to be seen more frequently in days prior to the pertussis immunisation.

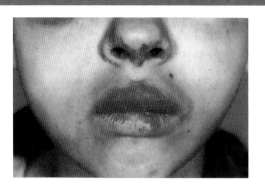

Fig 5.17

A 10-year-old girl presents with this vasculitic facial rash which has been worsening over several months. On examination in addition to the facial rash, she is found to have stigmata of chronic liver disease with spider naevi, leuconychia and mild clubbing. She also has a 7 cm spleen palpable, though only a firm liver edge. Her LFTs are as follows:

Bilirubin 35 µmol/l
ALT 185 U/l
AST 212 U/l
GGT 24 U/l
ALP 400 U/l
Albumin 36 g/l

What are the most likely diagnoses?

SELECT *TWO* ANSWERS ONLY

 i. Gilbert's syndrome
 ii. Wilson's disease
 iii. Autoimmune hepatitis
 iv. SLE
 v. Haemochromatosis
 vi. Biliary cirrhosis

ANSWERS TO CASE 5.17

ii. Wilson's disease

iii. Autoimmune hepatitis

The differential diagnosis includes autoimmune hepatitis and Wilson's disease (α-1 antitrypsin deficiency/chronic hepatitis infections should also be considered).

Additionally, it is important to note whether there is a family history of autoimmune disease.

Other factors which should be sought from the history include the medical history of the patient, any drug history, a history of deteriorating school performance, etc., and any exposure to i.v. blood or blood products.

Further investigations may include:

- Hepatitis serology

For Wilson's disease:

- slit lamp examination for Kaiser–Fleischer rings
- plasma caeruloplasmin
- urinary copper before and after a penicillamine challenge
- liver biopsy with measurement of liver copper concentration

For autoimmune hepatitis:

- auto-antibodies including antinuclear antibody (ANA)
- anti-smooth muscle (SMA) and anti-liver-kidney microsomal antibody (LKM-1)
- serum immunoglobulins
- liver biopsy

To exclude α-1 antitrypsin deficiency and chronic hepatitis viral infection:

- α-1 antitrypsin level and phenotype

It is important to monitor patients for development of acute liver failure. A rising bilirubin, an increasing prothrombin time and a falling serum albumin may all indicate failing liver function and the need for possible transplantation.

The most common causes for chronic liver disease presenting in previously healthy older children are autoimmune hepatitis and Wilson's disease. Differentiating between the two conditions can be difficult.

In autoimmune hepatitis, there is a 75% female preponderance, 20% have another autoimmune disease and 40% have a history of autoimmune disease in a first-degree relative. The aminotransferases are variably raised but the alkaline phosphatase tends to be normal. Type 1 characteristically has ANA and SMA positivity and type 2 has LKM-1 positivity. The diagnosis also depends on excluding other disorders, especially Wilson's disease. If coagulation allows, a liver biopsy should be performed to aid both diagnosis and assessment of the degree of inflammation and fibrosis. Cirrhosis is present in ~70% at diagnosis. Recurrence of the disease occurs in approximately 25% after transplantation.

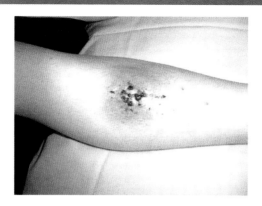

Fig 5.18

A 12-year-old girl, recently diagnosed with Crohn's disease had been commenced on appropriate treatment and, at outpatient review, her symptoms had improved. However, 6 weeks later, she developed exquisitely painful lesions in both axillae. She was given antibiotics with no improvement, and new lesions emerged on her arms and shins as shown.

What are these lesions?

SELECT THE *BEST* ANSWER

i. Kaposi's sarcoma
ii. Dermatitis herpetiformis
iii. Acanthosis nigrans
iv. Pyoderma gangrenosum
v. Erythema nodosum
vi. Necrobiosis lipoidica

ANSWER TO CASE 5.18

iv. Pyoderma gangrenosum

The lesions are pyoderma gangrenosum. The cause of this is not clear. Many associations with systemic disease have been described including inflammatory bowel disease, rheumatoid arthritis, leukaemia and chronic active hepatitis. Twenty per cent of patients have a history of trauma. Up to one-third of cases have no systemic illness. Pyoderma gangrenosum has the same prevalence in girls and boys, and in children has a mean age of onset of 10.2 years. The lesion often begins as a pustule which ruptures forming an ulcer with a mucopurulent base. They heal with a characteristic cribiform pattern of scarring. The most common site is the lower limbs. Histopathologic appearances vary and are usually not helpful in confirming the diagnosis.

The management of pyoderma gangrenosum is difficult. Topical and intralesional treatment is disappointing. Systemic steroids are the first-line therapy. Other immunosuppressive agents such as azathioprine or cyclosporin are frequently required, and some authors report satisfactory results with thalidomide.

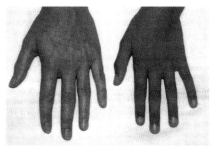 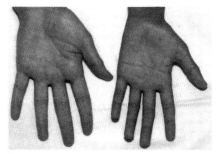

a   b

Fig 5.19

An 11-year-old girl was brought to hospital by ambulance. She had had 2 days of abdominal pain, vomited twice, slight headache and mild fever. She had become increasingly lethargic and slept during the day. When she awoke, she was confused, disorientated and unable to move. She had no previous medical problems, and had not travelled abroad since a holiday to Greece a year before, from which she had retained a suntan.

On examination, airway and breathing were normal, heart rate was 135 bpm, capillary refill was 4 s and blood pressure was 88/64 mmHg. GCS was 13 and temperature was 38.0°C. There were no localising signs of infection, including no meningism. Fundoscopy was normal.

Investigations were as follows: Hb 14.8 g/dl, WBC 13.7 × 10⁹/l, neutrophils 10.3 × 10⁹/l, platelets 307 × 10⁹/l, CRP 8 mg/l, Na 119 mmol/l, K 5.9 mmol/l, urea 6.6 mmol/l, creatinine 70 mmol/l, Ca 2.46 mmol/l, ALP 234 mmol/l, glucose 2.0 mmol/l.

Cranial CT, and CSF pressure, chemistry and microscopy were normal.

A full septic screen was performed. Figure 15.19.a and b show her hand (on the right, next to her older sister's for comparison).

What is most likely diagnosis?

SELECT *ONE* ANSWER ONLY
   i. Addison's disease
  ii. Waterhouse–Friederichson syndrome
 iii. SIADH (syndrome of inappropriate ADH secretion)
 iv. Water intoxication
   v. Acute renal failure
 vi. Cerebral infection (with associated salt wasting)
 vii. Conn's syndrome
viii. Bartter syndrome

ANSWER TO CASE 5.19

i. Addison's disease

The hyponatraemia is striking. The differential diagnosis includes the syndromes of inappropriate antidiuretic hormone secretion or cerebral salt wasting (secondary to intracranial infection), and water intoxication. However, the skin tanning and the hypoglycaemia suggest chronic adrenal failure and an Addisonian crisis precipitated by an infection.

Causes of *acute* adrenal insufficiency include adrenal destruction, e.g. haemorrhage due to birth trauma and Waterhouse–Fridierichson syndrome (sepsis and collapse, often associated with meningococcaemia). However, acute causes would not give skin pigmentation.

Initial management involves circulatory support with fluid boluses and inotropes if required, glucose, antibiotics for possible infection, and corticosteroids (with adequate sodium replacement, mineralocorticoids are not needed acutely).

Synacthen test (this must wait 12 h after a dose of hydrocortisone) results were as follows:
Cortisol at time
  0 min − 75 nmol/l
  30 min − 85 nmol/l
  60 min − 88 nmol/l

The absence of a rise confirms Addison's disease.

Investigations for the cause are also needed:
  auto-antibodies
  long-chain fatty acids (for adrenoleucodystrophy)
  CXR
  tuberculin test for tuberculosis

TB was the most common cause of adrenal failure in the 1950s. Auto-immune failure is now much more common. There are associations with other auto-immune conditions including hypothyroidism, hypoparathyroidism, mucocutaneous candidiasis, diabetes mellitus, cirrhosis and alopecia, but these can remain subclinical. Low T4 with raised TSH levels are common at presentation, but often correct rapidly with glucocorticoid treatment without thyroxine. Auto-antibody tests could encompass adrenal, thyroid, pituitary gland, coeliac, gastric parietal cell, antinuclear antibody, liver microsomal, smooth muscle and mitochondrial antibodies.

Treatment is with hydrocortisone and fludrocortisone. A mild androgenic preparation may improve libido and pubic hair growth in adolescent and adult women, but puberty is usually normal in timing and progression.

Other important aspects of long-term management include a "Medic Alert" bracelet, steroid card, information sheet and booklet about what to do when unwell, information to local A&E, and teaching the technique for emergency i.m. hydrocortisone injection.

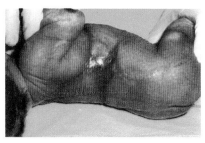

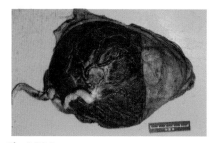

Fig 5.20.A

Fig 5.20.B

This term baby was growth retarded at birth and had this skin lesion. The pregnancy had been normal apart from maternal smoking.

What is the skin lesion shown?

SELECT *ONE* ANSWER ONLY

i. Congenital scleroderma
ii. Staphylococcal infection
iii. Congenital CMV
iv. Epidermolysis bullosa
v. Aplasia cutis congenita

ANSWER TO CASE 5.20

v. Aplasia cutis congenita (ACC)

Aplasia cutis congenita (ACC) is a rare disorder characterised by localised absence of skin at birth. This baby had a large area of symmetric aplasia cutis congenita affecting the parietal scalp on both sides, both thighs, both scapular areas and a band running across the midline of his back. This was treated conservatively with flamazine dressings, followed by hydrocortisone 1% over granulating areas and then simple jelonet and gauze. Skin grafting was not needed.

In the classification of ACC as proposed by Frieden et al, type V is related to the presence of a fetus papyraceous (see photo) or placental infarcts. In this case, the pregnancy was initially a twin pregnancy but one twin died at 11 weeks. The aetiology is thought to be placental transfer of emboli or thromboplastic material through vascular shunts. It is hypothesised that this precipitates DIC in the fetus, with a resultant hyper-coagulable state due to relative fetal antithrombin III deficiency. The skin defects are probably as a result of congenital vascular disruption secondary to embolisation. The reason for the characteristic symmetrical distribution is not known.

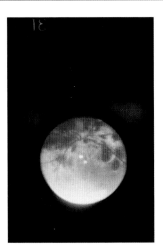

Fig 5.21

A 4-month-old boy was brought to casualty. His grandmother had found him unwell and "breathing funny" and called an ambulance. She said he was asleep when she arrived to baby-sit whilst his mother went out. He had apparently taken a full feed just before she arrived, but she found him unwell an hour later. Paramedics found him pale and obtunded and had noticed facial twitching.

On examination, he was pale and drowsy with a capillary refill time of 3 s and oxygen saturation of 88%. He was resuscitated and stabilised. Examination of his fundus was as shown and additional investigations gave the following results:

Hb 8.8 g/dl
WBC 22.4 × 10^9/l (neutrophils 30%, lymphocytes 68%, monocytes 2%)
platelets 780 × 10^9/l
CRP 86 mg/l
blood sugar 7.1 mmol/l
CSF examination – blood stained CSF (protein 0.64 mg/l, sugar 3.2 mmol/l)
CSF microscopy (WBC 3/mm³, RBC 1600/mm³, no organisms seen)

a. What is the most likely diagnosis?
   SELECT *ONE* ANSWER ONLY
   i. Meningococcal meningitis
   ii. Herpes encephalitis
   iii. Inflicted head injury
   iv. Aspiration pneumonia
   v. Urinary tract infection

b. Which one of the following is *not* necessary once the baby is stabilised?
   SELECT *ONE* ANSWER ONLY
   i. Skeletal survey
   ii. Coagulation screen
   iii. CT head
   iv. CT thorax
   v. Examination of siblings
   vi. Involvement of social services

a. iii. Inflicted head injury
b. iv. CT thorax

Inflicted head injury is an acute paediatric and neurosurgical emergency. Retinal haemorrhages are characteristically present, and ophthalmic examination is essential in any acutely unwell young child. The first priority is to resuscitate, stabilise and make appropriate referrals. Until the diagnosis is confirmed the baby should have a full septic screen and be treated with i.v. antibiotics. The parents should be contacted and interviewed. Associated injuries may include skull fractures, rib fractures and metaphyseal fractures of long bones. This type of abuse may be associated with a family under great stress, and other siblings need paediatric evaluation. Inflicted head injury carries significant mortality and morbidity, and clinicians should consider this possibility in all sick small infants with sudden neurological deterioration.

Further steps that may be required include care of airway and breathing possibly involving an anaesthetist; volume replacement, initially human albumin or plasma followed by a blood transfusion if necessary (clotting screen prior to transfusion). Urgent transfer to a paediatric intensive care unit should be considered. A thorough external examination for other signs suggestive of non-accidental injury should be performed, and an urgent CT scan of the brain with neurosurgical involvement as indicated. CT might reveal subdural haematomas, cerebral oedema, contusions, intracerebral haemorrhage, midline shift and acute hydrocephalus depending on timing and severity of injury.

A skeletal survey needs to be organised once the child is stabilised, and this will need repeating after 2 weeks (a single X-ray does not exclude injury). This might reveal skull fractures, rib fractures and metaphyseal fractures of long bones depending on timing and severity of injury. In some units bone scans are no longer routinely recommended in cases of child abuse.

There must be urgent contact with the parents to explain the situation, and early involvement of the child protection team. Arrangements need to be made with social services for evaluation of siblings, and moving to a place of safety if necessary.

The prognosis of these babies is very variable. Many will suffer long-term disability. Those most affected may show severe learning difficulties, cerebral atrophy and microcephaly, visual impairment, seizure disorders or cerebral palsy.

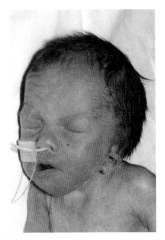

Fig 5.22.A

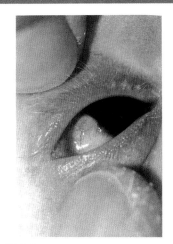

Fig 5.22.B

A baby girl was born at 30 weeks' gestation following prolonged rupture of the membranes from 25 weeks' gestation. She was in good condition at birth and developed no respiratory distress. She was noted to have an asymmetrical facial appearance and on closer inspection was found to have an epibulbar dermoid.

What is the diagnosis?

SELECT *ONE* ANSWER ONLY

  i. CHARGE association
  ii. Alagille syndrome
  iii. Treacher–Collins syndrome
  iv. Klippel–Feil abnormality
  v. Goldenhar syndrome
  vi. Pierre–Robin sequence

ANSWER TO CASE 5.22

v. Goldenhar syndrome

The photo shows a nasogastric tube in situ, an abnormal left ear, hypoplasia of the left side of the face, and a left facial nerve palsy. Closer inspection of the eye revealed an epibulbar dermoid.

Hemifacial microsomia, facio-auriculo-vertebral spectrum and Goldenhar syndrome are often used synonymously to describe this constellation of disorders affecting the jaw, mouth and ear unilaterally. Abnormalities of the eye (characteristically epibulbar dermoids) and vertebrae also occur. It generally occurs sporadically, although autosomal dominant and recessive patterns of inheritance have been described.

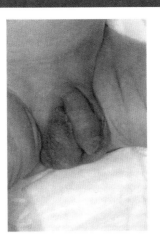

Fig 5.23

A 14-day-old baby was referred by his GP with a history of poor feeding and vomiting. He had been born at term following a normal pregnancy, weighing 3700 g. He was the first child of young parents. On examination, he weighed 3400 g and was lethargic and approximately 5% dehydrated. He was jaundiced and had oral and perineal candidiasis. His pulse was 150, BP 88/40. The appearance of his genitalia is shown. His initial electrolytes showed:

Na 115 mmol/l
K 6.7 mmol/l
Urea 11.8 mmol/l
Creatinine 117 mmol/l
Glucose 4.8 mmol/l

a. What is *not* required in the immediate management?
SELECT *ONE* ANSWER ONLY
  i. i.v. fluid rehydration with normal saline
 ii. i.v. fludrocortisone
iii. i.v. hydrocortisone
 iv. Regular blood glucose and blood pressure measurement
  v. Regular electrolyte measurements (4-6 hourly)

b. What investigations will confirm the diagnosis?
SELECT *TWO* ANSWERS ONLY
  i. Synacthen test
 ii. 21-hydroxyprogesterone (21-OHP)
iii. 17-hydroxyprogesterone (17-OHP)
 iv. Renin
  v. Cholesterol

ANSWERS TO CASE 5.23

a. ii. i.v. fluidrocortisone
b. iii. 17-hydroxyprogesterone (17-OHP)
   iv. Renin

The likely diagnosis here is congenital adrenal hyperplasia (CAH). This baby has presented in a salt-losing crisis, he has a rugose, pigmented scrotum and a large phallus, all consistent with a diagnosis of CAH. Classical CAH is due to a deficiency of the adrenal steroid 21-hydroxylase enzyme in 90% of cases. Affected female infants may be born with genital ambiguity of varying degrees; however, males have normal external genitalia and the diagnosis may not be obvious at birth. Those with deficient aldosterone production may therefore present with renal salt wasting and plasma volume loss with hyperkalaemia, which can lead to vascular collapse, shock and death. Dehydration from salt loss may occur as early as weeks 1-4 of life and this occurs in up to 75% of all cases of classical CAH. Those who do not present with a salt wasting crisis may present later with progressive virilisation.

In classical 21-OH deficiency, baseline 17-OHP concentrations are diagnostic, and renin will be elevated. Urinary steroid profiles should also be checked which will demonstrate the level of the enzyme block in the other forms of CAH.

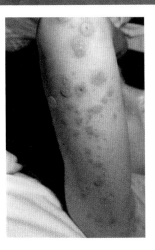

Fig 5.24

A 12-year-old girl was referred to the hospital by her GP with a widespread blistering rash. There was a 2-week history of cough and flu-like symptoms which had been treated with amoxycillin. The rash, which was itchy, started on her hands and then spread to the axillae, thighs, buttocks and arms. On examination, she was apyrexial, with a rash, but otherwise well. The rash was also present in her mouth and on her genitalia, palms and soles.

The girl was reviewed by the dermatologist who suggested two investigations as new crops of blisters continued to appear over the next few days.

On obtaining the results of the investigations, the dermatologist recommended treatment with dapsone or sulphamethoxypyridazine.

What do you think was the final diagnosis?

SELECT *ONE* ANSWER ONLY
  i. Bullous pemphigoid
  ii. Chronic bullous disease of childhood
  iii. Staphylococcal scalded skin syndrome (SSSS)
  iv. Herpes simplex type 2
  v. Epidermolysis bullosa type II
  vi. Hand, foot and mouth disease

ANSWER TO CASE 5.24

ii. Chronic bullous disease of childhood

Differential diagnoses of a bullous eruption should include:
Erythema multiforme (Stevens–Johnson syndrome)
Generalized herpes simplex
Chronic bullous disease of childhood (linear IgA disease).

It is important to send blister fluid to virology for electron microscopy from any bullous or vesicular eruption. The dermatologists may also perform a skin biopsy (for immunofluorescence).

Chronic bullous disease of childhood is an acquired, probably autoimmune, disease with involvement of skin and mucous membranes. The single most important investigation is a biopsy of uninvolved skin which shows subepidermal blisters characterised by IgA antibodies reacting with the basement membrane zone of the skin which is detected by direct immunofluorescence. There is no definitive treatment for this condition, and therapy is aimed at controlling the disease. In our patient, dapsone was not used as the child's preexisting anaemia could have been worsened by haemolysis, which is a known side-effect of the drug.

In approximately 65% of children, the disease goes into remission but in others it may persist into adult life.

Chapter

CASE 6.1

A 6-week-old boy is referred to clinic because of floppiness. He was born at term by spontaneous vaginal delivery. Examination reveals dysmorphic facial features, hepatomegaly and extensive generalised hypotonia. His cardiovascular and respiratory examination is normal.

Results of metabolic investigations are:
Blood lactate 7 mmol/l
Arterial blood gas normal
Organic and amino acids normal
Piperocolic acid marginally raised
Serum ammonia 80 μmol/l
Serum glucose 2.5 mmol/l
VLCFA increased
Phytanic acid raised
Dihydroxyacetone phosphate acyl transferase decreased

a. What diagnosis do these results infer?
   SELECT *ONE* ANSWER ONLY
   i. Biotinidase deficiency
  ii. Zellweger syndrome
 iii. Urea cycle disorder
  iv. Moebius syndrome

b. Choose three associated features of this condition:
   SELECT *THREE* ANSWERS ONLY
   i. Cleft palate
  ii. Neonatal hypoglycaemia
 iii. Large anterior fontanelle
  iv. Talipes equinovarus
   v. Patent ductus arteriosus
  vi. Absent corpus callosum
 vii. Retinopathy
viii. Syndactyly
  ix. Deafness

ANSWERS TO CASE 6.1

a. ii. Zellweger syndrome
b. iii. Large anterior fontanelle
   vii. Retinopathy
   ix. Deafness

This baby has Zellweger syndrome. This is one of a group of 17 peroxisomal disorders. Others include infantile Refsum and neonatal adrenoleukodystrophy. All of them present in a similar fashion and the absolute diagnosis depends on biochemical analysis. The cardinal features are facial dysmorphism including paucity of facial movements, large anterior fontanelle, prominent forehead, broad nasal root and hypoplastic supraorbital ridges; hepatomegaly (80%); prenatal renal cortical cysts (70%); congenital sensorineural hearing impairment (90%); cataracts (70%); peripheral pigmentary retinopathy (40%); optic nerve hypoplasia (40%); calcific stippling of the patellae and synchondrosis of the acetabulum.

Diagnosis is by electroretinogram (abnormal in 85%), brainstem auditory evoked potentials and skeletal survey. Biochemical abnormalities are increased saturated VLCFA. C26:0 may be 5 times normal (0.33 mcg/ml). In addition, ratios of C24:0/C22:0 and C26:0/C22:0 are raised. Many gene mutations have been identified that cause abnormalities in peroxisome assembly and function.

CASE 6.2

You are asked to see a 24-hour-old male infant on the postnatal ward because he has small spots all over his body. He is feeding well and appears otherwise completely healthy.

On examination he has petechial spots over his face, trunk and limbs. He has no organomegaly or lymphadenopathy and the rest of the examination is normal.

FBC showed: Hb 15.7 g/dl, WCC 12.0×10^9/l and platelets 10×10^9/l.

What are the most likely diagnoses?

SELECT *TWO* ANSWERS ONLY

   i. Maternal idiopathic thrombocytopaenic purpura
  ii. Kasabach–Merritt syndrome
 iii. Congenital leukaemia
 iv. Congenital rubella
  v. Alloimmune thrombocytopaenic purpura
 vi. Traumatic petechiae
vii. Maternal anticonvulsant therapy

ANSWERS TO CASE 6.2

 i. Maternal idiopathic thrombocytopaenic purpura
 v. Alloimmune thrombocytopaenic purpura

Investigations should include checking the maternal platelet count and maternal antiplatelet antibodies.

Isolated thrombocytopaenia in the neonate is usually related to transplacental IgG from the mother.

Neonatal alloimmune thrombocytopaenia (NAIT) is similar to haemolytic disease of the newborn, with maternal antibodies crossing the placenta to destroy fetal cells.

NAIT is caused by maternal antibodies directed against fetal platelet antigens, inherited from the father, which cross and enter the fetal circulation. These antibody-covered platelets in the fetus or in the neonate are destroyed at an increased rate, leading to thrombocytopaenia and petechiae.

Human platelet antigen-1a (HPA-1a, formerly known as PL[A1]) is the most common antigen found in over 75% of cases.

NAIT with platelet counts <50 000/μl occurs in about 1 : 1000 births.

Management involves daily platelet counts and platelet transfusions if levels fall below 20–30 000/μl or if there is significant bleeding. Babies should be closely monitored for external and internal bleeding such as intracranial haemorrhage. The natural history of NAIT is that the thrombocytopaenia usually resolves within 3–4 weeks but can last up to 3 months. It is important that parents are counselled regarding future pregnancies.

Autoimmune neonatal thrombocytopaenia is usually seen in babies whose mothers have a history of idiopathic thrombocytopaenic purpura (ITP).

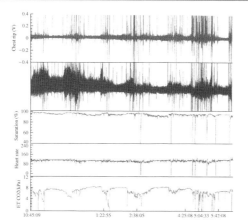

Fig 6.3

A 2-month-old baby boy was presented to casualty, collapsed. His mother's pregnancy had been normal, as was his birth. The examination after his resuscitation was normal. He was admitted to the paediatric intensive care unit. Extensive investigations at the time were normal. He was easy to ventilate and quickly weaned from the ventilator.

The following night he collapsed on the ward and required reventilating. An arterial blood gas 1 h after reventilating showed: pH 7.35, PO_2 13.0 kPa, PCO_2 5.9 kPa and base excess 3.7 mmol/l. The sleep study is shown. When he was not ventilated an early morning capillary gas showed a raised PCO_2.

What is the most likely diagnosis?

SELECT *ONE* ANSWER ONLY
  i. Congenital myasthenia gravis
  ii. Congenital cystic adenomatoid malformation of the lung
  iii. Pulmonary hypertension
  iv. Bronchopulmonary dysplasia
  v. Duchenne muscular dystrophy
  vi. Ondine's curse

ANSWER TO CASE 6.3

vi. Ondine's curse

Diagnoses which must be considered when he deteriorates on weaning from the ventilator include partially treated sepsis, seizure, arrhythmia, inborn error of metabolism or a disorder of breathing control, e.g. Ondine's curse, also known as idiopathic congenital central hypoventilation syndrome (CCHS).

Investigations should include an early morning blood gas off the ventilator, 12-lead ECG, cranial imaging and a sleep study. Other investigations to be considered include bronchoscopy, ophthalmological opinion, echocardiogram and muscle biopsy.

The ease of ventilation and the dramatic response on two occasions in this case make the diagnosis of CCHS most likely.

This is confirmed by the sleep study – the chest and abdominal bands show a variable respiratory effort. When the effort is poor there is hypoxia and hypercarbia.

CCHS (Ondine's curse) is rare. It is the CO_2 level during or prior to the collapse that is important. This could be measured on a blood gas at the time or by a formal sleep study. A typical sleep study in CCHS shows episodes of hypoxia associated with hypercarbia and decreased chest and abdominal wall movement. The management of CCHS is lifelong overnight ventilation. CCHS is associated with Hirschsprung's disease, ophthalmological problems, ganglioneuroma, neuroblastoma, oesophageal dysmotility and heart rate variability.

An 8-year-old child was referred by his GP with a 6-week history of lethargy, secondary nocturnal enuresis, thirst and occasional vomiting. He showed normal growth and examination was unremarkable apart from possible pigmentation of his knuckles and umbilicus.

Initial investigations by the GP gave the following results:
Hb 14.5 g/dl
Na 131 mmol/l
K 5.3 mmol/l
Urea 11.1 mmol/l
Creatinine 65 µmol/l
Glucose 3.4 mmol/l
Thyroid function normal
Random cortisol 276 nmol/l (120-400)

a. What is the most likely diagnosis and what test would you do to confirm the diagnosis?
    SELECT THE BEST PAIR OF ANSWERS

a. Hypopituitarism   1. Chromosomes
b. Noonan syndrome   2. Echocardiogram
c. Cushing's syndrome   3. Short synacthen test
d. Kallman's syndrome   4. Cerebral MRI
e. Addison's disease   5. Insulin tolerance test

b. If this child had been found to have a low serum calcium, what other diagnosis would need to be considered?
    SELECT *ONE* ANSWER ONLY

 i. Hypercalcaemia
 ii. Hypophosphatasia
iii. Hypoparathyroidism
iv. Pseudohypoparathyroidism (PHP)
 v. Vitamin D dependent rickets

ANSWERS TO CASE 6.4

a. e. and 3. Addison's disease and short synacthen test
b. iii. Hypoparathyroidism

This child has Addison's disease (autoimmune adrenal failure), which can be confirmed by a short synacthen test. This was abnormal in the child showing a basal cortisol level of 180 nmol/l with no response to stimulation. Random cortisol levels are unhelpful in this situation as an elevated ACTH may maintain them in the normal range initially.

The diagnosis can be confirmed by the presence of anti-adrenal cytoplasmic antibodies.

If there was associated hypocalcaemia found, type I autoimmune polyendocrinopathy also needs to be considered. In this disorder, hypoparathyroidism precedes the development of Addison's disease and is also associated with mucocutaneous candidiasis.

A 20-month-old boy was scalded by hot coffee spilling onto his upper chest, causing a 3% body surface burn. A&E staff assessed the burn as mainly superficial partial thickness. He was treated with simple analgesia and a silicone-gauze dressing and discharged. The following day he developed a fever, diarrhoea and vomiting. That evening he attended his local GP out-of-hours service and was referred to hospital. At triage his pulse was 165 bpm, respiratory rate 36/min and blood pressure 100/65 mmHg; he had a temperature of 39.1°C. He was pale, drowsy, with mild clinical dehydration but no rash, focal neurological signs or neck stiffness. His burn looked clean with no sign of cellulitis. Initial laboratory studies showed a WBC of 5.2 × 10^9/l, platelet count of 232 × 10^9/l and normal plasma glucose. U&Es supported mild dehydration: Na 132 mmol/l, K 2.5 mmol/l, urea 12 mmol/l. He was started on i.v. fluids. He developed progressive circulatory failure, reduced urine output and a high fever. His WBC rose to 25 × 10^9/l, platelets fell to 83 × 10^9/l, and he developed a coagulopathy. His U&Es showed marked worsening of his hyponatraemia, hypokalaemia and uraemia, and LFTs became abnormal.

What is the most likely diagnosis?

SELECT *ONE* ANSWER ONLY

   i. Staphylococcal scalded skin syndrome
  ii. Toxic shock syndrome
 iii. Kawasaki syndrome
 iv. Toxic epidermal necrolysis
  v. Stevens–Johnson syndrome
 vi. Necrotising fasciitis

ANSWER TO CASE 6.5

ii. Toxic shock syndrome (TSS)

This is a potentially life-threatening exotoxin-mediated disease caused by *Staphylococcus aureus* or *Streptococcus pyogenes*. The staphylococcal exotoxin, toxic shock syndrome toxin-1 (TSST-1), diffuses into the blood and causes the illness in the absence of tissue invasion by staphylococci. Low or absent levels of antiTSST-1 antibodies may indicate susceptibility to the illness. Management involves intensive care with aggressive fluid resuscitation, i.v. antibiotic therapy (cefotaxime and flucloxacillin), vasopressors and immunoglobulin therapy. TSS is an uncommon but well-established complication of even relatively minor burns in children. In most cases there is a prodromal period with fever (>38.9°C), myalgia, headache, vomiting and diarrhoea before the onset of hypotension and multiorgan failure. A generalised macular erythematous rash develops after a few days. In the recovery phase there is desquamation of the palms and soles, fingers and toes. Parents should be advised to seek professional advice if their child develops a feverish illness after a burn injury.

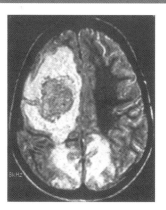

Fig 6.6

A 6-year-old girl presented with a low-grade pyrexia, poor appetite, painful elbows and ankles, abdominal pain and diarrhoea. On examination, she had flushed cheeks, a papular itchy rash on her right arm, an ejection systolic murmur and minimal swelling and tenderness of the affected ankle joints. She failed to improve with her initial management but on day 3 developed a characteristic rash. She also had blood and protein in her urine and had developed mild hypertension. She began to improve spontaneously over the next few days but subsequently went on to develop some uncommon but serious complications of this illness (see Fig. 6.6).

a. What conditions would you include in your initial differential diagnosis?
   SELECT *THREE* APPROPRIATE ANSWERS
   i. Scarlet fever
   ii. Henoch–Schönlein purpura
   iii. Nephrotic syndrome
   iv. Rheumatic fever
   v. Lyme disease
   vi. Kawasaki's disease
   vii. Vasculitis
   viii. Systemic juvenile chronic arthritis
   ix. Measles
   x. Subacute bacterial endocarditis

b. The scan illustrates an extremely rare complication of this condition. What does it show?
   SELECT *ONE* ANSWER ONLY
   i. Cerebral haematoma
   ii. Cerebral abscess
   iii. Cerebral tumour
   iv. Meningitis

ANSWERS TO CASE 6.6

a. ii. Henoch–Schönlein purpura (HSP)
    iv. Rheumatic fever
    viii. Systemic juvenile chronic arthritis
b. i. Cerebral haematoma

Initial differential diagnosis should include bacterial sepsis, viral infection, rheumatic fever, Henoch–Schönlein purpura, systemic juvenile chronic arthritis. By day three the diagnosis of Henoch–Schönlein purpura should have been made.

The MRI scan shows a large right fronto-parietal haematoma surrounded by oedema.

Sixty per cent of children with HSP will have some degree of nephritis, from microscopic haematuria to a full-blown nephritic picture. Those that need nephrology follow-up include those with persistent moderate proteinuria, those who present with an acute nephritic or nephritic-nephrotic picture, or those with progressive renal impairment.

Of those with microscopic haematuria only, almost 100% are likely to have normal GFR and BP at 10 years. In contrast, of those who are nephritic, 40% will have end-stage renal disease at 10 years and only 20% will have normal renal function.

CASE 6.7

A 4-year-old presents to casualty with a limp. He is thought to have an irritable hip. After a normal hip X-ray, he is discharged. He continues to have intermittent hip and back pain and is seen by the GP who follows him up for anaemia. The anaemia fails to respond to 4 weeks of haematinics and he is referred to the nearest hospital. He has a left-sided limp on admission and complains of pain in the right leg. His Hb is 7.5 g/dl. There are no other clinical findings.

a. What investigations would you do next?
    SELECT *FOUR* ANSWERS ONLY
    i. Repeat hip X-ray
    ii. MRI hip
    iii. FBC and film
    iv. Erythrocyte sedimentation rate
    v. CXR
    vi. Left knee X-ray
    vii. X-ray lumbar spine
    viii. MRI spine
    ix. Bone scan
    x. Skeletal survey
    xi. B12 and folate
    xii. Bone marrow aspiraton

b. On reviewing the first X-ray, there is a small lytic lesion in the femoral head. What differentials would you initially consider?
    SELECT THE *THREE* MOST APPROPRIATE ANSWERS
    i. Haemophagocytic lymphohistiocytosis
    ii. Osteomyelitis
    iii. Histiocytosis
    iv. Avascular necrosis
    v. Astrocytoma
    vi. Neuroblastoma
    vii. Slipped upper femoral epiphysis
    viii. McCune-Albright syndrome
    ix. Albright's hereditary osteodystrophy
    x. Collapsed congenital bone cyst

ANSWERS TO CASE 6.7

a.   i. Repeat hip X-ray
   iii. FBC and film
   iv. Erythrocyte sedimentation rate
   v. CXR
b. ii. Osteomyelitis
   iii. Histiocytosis
   vi. Neuroblastoma

History of pain in a child should always be regarded with caution, particularly persistent and localised. Backache is never normal in a child. Failure to respond to haematinics (for anaemia) raised questions of aetiology. History should include bleeding tendency, fever or sweating, loss of weight and diarrhoea. FBC, differential and blood film, and CRP/ESR should be checked. Blood cultures, CXR and a repeat hip X-ray should be done. Differentials of lytic bone lesions include osteomyelitis, histiocytosis, giant cell tumour, malignant tumours, neuroblastoma, peripheral primitive neuroectodermal tumour, and Ewing's sarcoma. Abdominal USS revealed a large, clinically non-palpable, retroperitoneal mass. AXR revealed widespread calcification. CXR was normal. Urine catecholamines were markedly raised. A CT scan confirmed the mass and its extension: invasion of the bone marrow with tumour cells. A diagnostic biopsy showed neuroblastoma. Bone scan and MIBG revealed extensive bone metastases.

Neuroblastoma has myriad modalities of presentation. It can arise from any site along the sympathetic nervous chain. Tumours may arise in the abdomen, adrenals, thoracic or cervical areas. Metastatic extension is lymphatic and haematogenous. The latter invades the bone marrow and results in anaemia. Bone metastases cause pain and lead to limping in young children. Due to the type of catecholamine metabolites released, hypertension is uncommon. Spontaneous bleeding into these tumours may herald severe abdominal pain. High thoracic and cervical masses can be associated with Horner's syndrome, superior vena cava syndrome and cord compression. Retrobulbar and orbital infiltration with tumour may result in proptosis and periorbital ecchymoses. Skin involvement is exclusive to infants and presents as non-tender bluish subcutaneous nodules. Paraneoplastic syndromes associated with neuroblastoma include opsomyoclonus or cerebellar ataxia, and intractable secretory diarrhoea associated with hypokalaemia and dehydration.

CASE 6.8

A 13-year-old girl has been diagnosed with Turner's syndrome following investigations into her short stature and mild learning difficulties. She is below the 0.4th centile for height on a normal growth chart and on the 75th centile on a Turner's growth chart. Initial investigations reveal normal thyroid function, antigliadin screen, serum urea and electrolytes, bone profile, haemoglobin A1C, cholesterol and triglycerides, with markedly elevated gonadotrophin levels, low oestradiol and very small ovaries on pelvic ultrasound. Her growth velocity is 1.5 cm/year giving a projected adult height of 145 cm (4' 9"), so growth hormone therapy is commenced with the intention to introduce oestrogen therapy later. One month after starting therapy, she develops intermittent right-sided frontal headache lasting 1-2 min with blurring of her vision. Her optic discs are swollen, visual fields are full to confrontation and neurological examination is unremarkable. A CT brain scan is normal. A lumbar puncture is performed with the following CSF results:

cytospin no cells seen
protein 0.27 g/l
glucose 3 mmol/l
microscopy 3 RBC and 0 WBC/HPF
opening pressure 22 cmH$_2$O

What is the most likely diagnosis?

SELECT *ONE* ANSWER ONLY
i. Venous sinus thrombosis
ii. Leukaemia
iii. Benign intracranial hypertension
iv. Hypoparathyroidism
v. Space-occupying lesion
vi. Viral encephalitis

ANSWER TO CASE 6.8

iii. Benign intracranial hypertension

This girl has developed benign intracranial hypertension. This can be idiopathic but is also reported as a rare side-effect of growth hormone (GH) therapy.

At the time of the lumbar puncture, CSF should be drained until the CSF opening pressure is normal for her age (approximately 15 cm H_2O). GH therapy should be discontinued. Benign intracranial hypertension is not a "benign" condition and the patient is at risk of visual deterioration and eventual blindness without appropriate management. Treatment is with acetazolamide, regular monitoring of serum potassium levels and supplementation as required. Treatment needs careful co-ordination with ophthalmological review. If headaches persist and eye signs do not improve, fortnightly lumbar punctures and steroid therapy may be necessary or in some cases a shunt procedure.

Other diagnoses which need to be excluded include:
- connective tissue diseases, e.g. systemic lupus erythematosus
- leukaemia
- venous sinus thrombosis, especially with otitis media or sinusitis (Gradenigo's syndrome).
- endocrine problems, such as diabetes mellitis, hyperadrenalism, hyperthyroidism and hypoparathyroidism (already considered in this case)

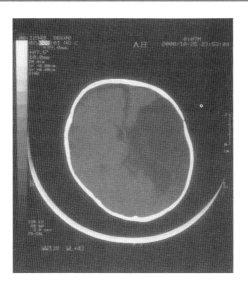

Fig 6.9.1

An 8-month-old baby boy presented initially with clustered episodes (over 2-3 min, several times a day) of right-sided twitching of the face and body, with head and eye deviation to the right. He was the firstborn twin (33 weeks' gestation by Caesarean section for antepartum haemorrhage), Apgar scores for the twins were 7 and 9 at 1 and 5 min, respectively. Twin-to-twin transfusion was suspected antenatally and regular scans were performed. Some amniotic fluid was drained from the amniotic sac of twin 1 on one occasion but no transfusions were given. His weight was on the 50th centile (twin 2 on the 25th) but he was not plethoric at birth. Both twins were admitted to the neonatal unit after delivery and required oxygen therapy briefly. Developmental history revealed that he smiled at 3 months, was cooing and laughing, reaching mostly with the left hand but not yet rolling or sitting. On examination, his head circumference is on the 50th centile and weight on the 98th centile, he had slight head lag, subtle facial asymmetry and a likely right visual field deficit. There was a paucity of movement on the right side but no difference in tone or tendon reflexes. He subsequently developed abnormal movements involving trunk flexion and extension of his upper limbs. An EEG was obtained which showed chaotic and continuous abnormal background of very high voltage with random slow waves and spikes.

a. What is the most likely diagnosis?
   SELECT *ONE* ANSWER ONLY
   i. Congenital toxoplasmosis infection
   ii. Acute disseminated encephalomyelitis
   iii. Cerebral palsy
   iv. Hypoxic ischaemic encephalopathy
   v. West's syndrome
   vi. Rett's syndrome

b. What lesion is seen on the CT shown?
   SELECT *ONE* ANSWER ONLY
   i. Anencephaly
   ii. Left sided subdural haemorrhage
   iii. Hydrancephaly
   iv. Periventricular leukomalacia with left ventricular dilatation
   v. Left porencephalic cyst
   vi. Lissencephaly

ANSWERS TO CASE 6.9

a. v. West's syndrome
b. v. Left porencephalic cyst

This child has delayed motor milestones. Persistent head lag at this age is abnormal and he would be expected to be rolling, although not sitting. The clear hand preference at this age is abnormal and indicates a right hemiparesis. The most likely diagnosis here is West's syndrome with hypsarrhythmia on the EEG.

The CT shows a left porencephalic cyst, which has developed secondary to an infarct in the territory of the right middle cerebral artery, occurring in the antenatal period. A twin-to-twin transfusion was suspected in utero and the recipient would have been susceptible to vascular events, although this is more common when the donor twin has died in utero. Infarcts such as these also occur sporadically.

CASE 6.10

A 17-year-old girl with Down's syndrome is seen for review at her school. She has previously been healthy but required grommets as a young child because of conductive hearing problems. Her parents are concerned that she had dropped two clothing sizes over recent months; she was previously overweight. Her family and GP are aware that she has missed some of her recommended health screens, particularly the blood tests, because she is noncompliant with venepuncture. She is complaining of intermittent abdominal pain but there is no bowel or urinary disturbance. An abdominal ultrasound was normal, as was urinalysis. On examination, height is on the 5th centile and weight on the 10th centile on the Down's syndrome growth chart. She has a slightly high resting pulse rate and a short mid-systolic murmur heard at the mid/upper sternal edge which did not radiate anywhere or vary in posture. Blood pressure was 100/70 mmHg. Otherwise, examination was unremarkable. There is no relevant family history.

a. Which medical conditions are more prevalent in individuals with Down's syndrome?
   SELECT *FIVE* ANSWERS ONLY
   i. Hyperthyroidism
  ii. Hypothyroidism
 iii. Sensorineural hearing loss
 iv. Fallots tetralogy
  v. Bronchiectasis
 vi. Atrial fibrillation
 vii. Asthma
viii. Crohn's disease
 ix. Hypopituitarism
  x. Scoliosis

Blood was sent for thyroid function with the following results:
   Free T4 48.2
   Free T3 12
   TSH <0.02
   Antithyroid peroxidase 390 K/l (<32.0).

b. What is the most likely diagnosis?
   SELECT *ONE* ANSWER ONLY
   i. Grave's disease
  ii. Congenital hypothyroidism
 iii. Acquired hypothyroidism
 iv. Hypopituitarism
  v. Hashimoto's thyroiditis

ANSWERS TO CASE 6.10

a.　i. Hyperthyroidism
　　ii. Hypothyroidism
　　iii. Sensorineural hearing loss
　　iv. Fallots tetralogy
　　x. Scoliosis
b.　i. Grave's disease

The following conditions are more prevalent in Down's syndrome:

- Cardiac: 40-60% of babies with Down's syndrome have congenital heart disease and 50% of these have atrio-ventricular septal defect. Other abnormalities that are more prevalent in these children include Fallot's tetralogy and various combinations of VSD/ASD.
- Orthopaedic: cervical spine instability, hip subluxation/dislocation, patellar instability, scoliosis, metatarsus varus and pes planus. Laxity of the transverse ligament of C1 or dysplasia of C1/C2 can predispose to dislocation or subluxation of the atlantoaxial joint with potentially catastrophic complications. There are no screening methods to predict who of the Down's population is at risk. Sporting activities should not be restricted if no clinical symptoms are present. Particular attention is needed when manipulating the neck of an unconscious child.
- Ears, nose and throat: >50% of children with Down's syndrome have hearing loss. Conductive losses are more common than sensorineural losses, and tend to persist into adolescence and adult life. Sensorineural losses, particularly presbyacusis, occur more with advancing age. Upper airway obstruction and infection are also more prevalent.
- Ophthalmological: refractive errors occur in approximately 70% of individuals with Down's syndrome. Congenital cataracts, nystagmus, squint, glaucoma, keratoconus, blepharitis and blocked nasolacrimal ducts are also more common.
- Endocrine: thyroid dysfunction, commonly hypothyroidism and less commonly hyperthyroidism is increasingly prevalent with advancing age. Uncompensated hypothyroidism is found in 10% of patients of school age. Growth failure may arise as a result of other chronic disease. Short stature is a feature of the condition and adapted centile charts are available. Diabetes is also more common.
- GI: 10% of children with Down's syndrome have congenital malformations such as atresia of the jejunum, duodenum, oesophagus and anus, annular pancreas and exomphalos. Coeliac disease and Hirschsprungs disease are also more prevalent; gastro-oesophageal reflux and oro-motor dysfunction can lead to feeding difficulties.
- Immunological: immunodeficiency and autoimmune problems such as arthropathy, vitiligo and alopecia are more common.
- Haematological: transient neonatal myeloproliferative states, leukaemia, neonatal polycythaemia and thrombocytopenia may be seen.
- Neuropsychiatric: infantile spasms, myoclonic epilepsies, autism and dementia (adults only) are more prevalent in this population.

The diagnosis here is Grave's disease. The management is initially carbimazole to render her euthyroid and then replacement thyroxine as necessary. This is generally discontinued after about 6 months and if relapse occurs, definitive treatment with radioactive iodine is given.

The following health checks are recommended by the UK Down's Syndrome Medical Interest Group:

- Thyroid function: birth to 6 weeks (routine neonatal screen), then thyroid function test including antibodies at 12 months, 3 years and then every second year or if clinically indicated. Annual dried blood spot TSH measurement using fingerprick blood may be available in some districts.
- Growth: length, weight and head circumference should be checked at any review appointment during the first year and then annually. Down's-specific charts should be used.

- Eye check: check for visual behaviour and cataract at birth, visual behaviour and squint at 6 and 12 months and from 2 years onwards, orthoptic examination, refraction and ophthalmological assessment every second year throughout life or when clinically indicated.
- Hearing: if locally available, neonatal screening should be arranged and full audiological review (hearing, impedance, otoscopy) subsequently at 6 months, yearly until 5 years and then every second year.
- Cardiovascular assessment: full assessment including echocardiogram should ideally be arranged in the first 6 weeks. The possibility of acquired heart disease should be considered at medical reviews for example secondary to upper airway obstruction.

Is it safe for a bottle-fed baby of 6 weeks to go swimming in the local chlorinated leisure centre?

SELECT *ONE* ANSWER ONLY

  i. No, because the baby has not yet received any polio vaccine and risks contracting poliomyelitis from a recently immunised child
 ii. No, because the baby has not yet received a full course of polio vaccine and risks contracting poliomyelitis from a recently immunised child
iii. No, because the baby has not yet received a full course of polio vaccine and risks contracting vaccine-associated poliomyelitis from a recently immunised child
 iv. Yes

ANSWER TO CASE 6.11

iv. Yes

Yes in chlorinated pools, but until the child has received a full course of polio vaccine, not in seawater, as it may be contaminated with sewage. There is no risk of an unimmunised child contracting vaccine-associated poliomyelitis from a recently immunised child if they are taken swimming, so recently immunised children may be taken swimming, even if they have been given oral polio vaccine.

An 8-week-old baby girl presented to hospital with bruising. She had small bruises over the left cheek, left lower back and left shin. The baby was an asylum seeker from Eastern Europe, housed in a bed-sit shared with her mother, both maternal grandparents and four maternal aunts/uncles with ages ranging from 2 to18 years. There was no history of trauma. The baby was fully breast fed and the mother was noted to be very thin. The baby weighed 3750 g (2nd centile). General examination was unremarkable except for the bruises.

The baby was investigated with FBC, coagulation screen, U+Es, bone chemistry and LFTs.

Blood results were as follows:

Hb 9.4 g/dl
WCC 11.1×10^9/l
Platelets 466×10^9/l
Total Ca 2.13 mmol/l
Corrected Ca 2.23 mmol/l
Phosphate 1.28 mmol/l
ALP 864 IU/l
Bilirubin 18 μmol/l
ALT 27 IU/l
Total protein 52 g/l

PT 18 s
APTT 36 s
Fibrinogen 1.8 g/l
Factor II 30% (34-102%)
Factor VIII 107% (50-150%)
Factor IX 13% (21-81%)
Factor X 30% (31-81%)
Factor XI 64% (50-150%)

What diagnoses are suggested by these results?

SELECT *TWO* ANSWERS ONLY

  i. Hyperparathyroidism
 ii. Non-accidental injury
iii. Vitamin D deficiency
 iv. Hypoparathyroidism
  v. Von Willebrand's disease
 vi. Haemophilia B
vii. Vitamin K deficiency

ANSWERS TO CASE 6.12

iii. Vitamin D deficiency
vii. Vitamin K deficiency

The history here raises the possibility of non-accidental injury (NAI). This should be considered in any infant presenting with unexplained bruising.

A skeletal survey and ophthalmologic referral for fundoscopy should be performed routinely in any infant with a suspected NAI. Children under the age of one year should also have a CT head.

However, the results here demonstrate vitamin K deficiency. Clotting factors II, VII, IX and X are vitamin K dependent. Vitamin K deficiency results in a prolonged PT and reduced assays of the dependent clotting factors. It is more common in breast-fed infants. It may present with easy bruising. In this case, oral vitamin K prophylaxis had been prescribed and dispensed, but was not given on account of communication difficulties.

The biochemical results are consistent with a diagnosis of vitamin D deficiency (rickets). Vitamin D levels in the fully breast-fed infant are dependent upon the nutritional state of the mother. In this case, the mother had nutritional vitamin D deficiency, accentuated by a reduction in exposure to sunlight. Vitamin D deficiency results in a raised alkaline phosphatase, low calcium and a low normal phosphate level. This baby had poorly mineralised bones on X-ray. Treatment is a course of alfacalcidol 25-50 ng/kg.

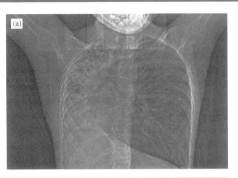

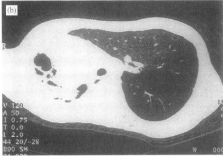

Fig 6.13.1

A 12-year-old girl complaining of chronic shortness of breath, poor exercise tolerance, and a long-standing cough productive of copious purulent sputum attends for a chest radiograph, after which a CT of the chest is performed. At the age of 8 years, she had a severe respiratory tract infection with pertussis. There was no other medical history of note.

What is the likely pathology in the right lung?

SELECT *ONE* ANSWER ONLY
  i. Wegener's granulomatosis
  ii Fibrosing alveolitis
 iii. Bronchiectasis
 iv. Legionnaire's disease
  v. Congenital pulmonary hypoplasia
 vi. Pneumocystis carinii pneumonia
 vii. Pneumatocoeles

ANSWER TO CASE 6.13

iii. Bronchiectasis

The chest radiograph demonstrates marked abnormality on the right with loss of volume and widespread ring shadows seen predominantly in the mid and upper zones. The mediastinum is shifted to the right and there is more confluent shadowing at the right base which probably represents consolidation as evidenced by the multiple air bronchograms seen. The left lung has herniated across the midline and appears to be of large volume consistent with a degree of air trapping. No focal consolidation or ring shadows are seen on the left.

The CT confirms the abnormalities on the right where ring and tubular air spaces can be seen. It is also noted that the right hemithorax is smaller than the left, consistent with a long-standing process. On the left, the CT shows considerable "mosaic attenuation" with the more posterior aspect of the left lung being of markedly lower attenuation (i.e. darker) than the anterior aspect. In addition, the darker lung has much fewer vessels per unit area, adding to the lower attenuation.

Given the history of chronic dyspnoea and a chronic productive cough, coupled with the findings on both chest radiography and CT of ring and tubular shadowing and ongoing consolidation, the most likely diagnosis is bronchiectasis.

Bronchiectasis usually originates in childhood and can be defined as irreversible dilatation of the bronchial tree, usually localised. The definition includes the term irreversible to exclude transient airway dilatation occasionally associated with pneumonia and atelectasis. There are numerous causes for bronchiectasis, the commonest being postinfectious (including viral, pertussis, allergic bronchopulmonary aspergillosis and tuberculosis), endoluminal bronchial obstruction (e.g. foreign body or mucoid impaction, seen particularly in patients with cystic fibrosis), ciliary dyskinesia (e.g. Kartagener syndrome), or secondary to longstanding immune compromise (e.g. chronic granulomatous disease of childhood). It is seen less nowadays than previously, due to improved antibiotic therapy, vaccines against measles and pertussis, and more effective physiotherapy. Postinfective bronchiectasis tends to be basally distributed in the lungs while that due to cystic fibrosis or immune deficiency is usually upper zone in distribution. The chest radiograph is occasionally normal in bronchiectasis (in approximately 7%, especially early in the disease) but usually demonstrates abnormalities including crowding of the bronchi, bronchial wall thickening, loss of definition of lung markings due to peribronchial fibrosis, and lobar loss of volume, especially at the bases, with compensatory emphysema of the upper lobes. End-stage changes include ring and tramline shadows (due to dilated bronchi seen end on and along their length, respectively) which can give rise to a honeycomb appearance, as seen in the mid- and upper zones in this case. Consolidation is a frequent complication, again as seen here. High-resolution CT (1 mm slices, either 10 or 20 mm apart) has become the radiological method of choice for the investigation of suspected bronchiectasis, as it is very sensitive to dilated bronchi. A bronchus should be of the same diameter as its accompanying pulmonary artery on CT; if the bronchus is dilated, the so-called "signet ring" appearance is produced. Other signs of bronchiectasis include the visualization of dilated bronchi more peripherally in the lung than usual, i.e. within 1 cm of the pleura. Cystic bronchiectasis may demonstrate air-fluid levels within the dilated bronchi. Contrast bronchography is rarely performed nowadays for the diagnosis of bronchiectasis but is occasionally used to delineate the extent of disease if surgery is considered.

A mosaic attenuation pattern as seen in the left lung, due to a combination of hypoperfusion and hypoventilation, has a number of causes, including chronic thromboembolic disease and asthma. However, in the context of a previous severe chest infection, the most likely underlying diagnosis is bronchiolitis obliterans. In this condition, endo- and peribronchiolar inflammation causes distal airway occlusion. In the developing lung this chronic hypoventilation gives rise to a decreased number of alveoli which are emphysematous, and hypoplasia of the pulmonary arteries supplying the affected segment, with resulting hypoperfusion. Aside from previous infections (including pertussis, viral and mycoplasma), other causes of bronchiolitis obliterans include toxic inhalation (ammonia and phosgene), foreign body inhalation, chronic graft vs host disease and post heart–lung transplant. A large percentage of cases, are, however, idiopathic.

CASE 6.14

A term neonate (3500 g) after an uneventful pregnancy and delivery, was found on the post-natal ward to be cyanotic (at 8 hours of age). He was initially put on CPAP and then ventilated.

Ventilation settings:
   CMV pressure 38/6, FiO_2 0.6
   SaO_2 50%
Rt radial arterial stab
   pH: 7.5
   PaO_2: 3 kPa
   $PaCO_2$: 3 kPa
   BE: 0
Normal 4-limb blood pressure
Normal perfusion

An umbilical arterial catheter (UAC) was inserted (12 cm) and bright red blood was seen on drawing back the syringe. A CXR was done to check the position of the UAC, showing mild patchy changes bilaterally; the tip of the UAC was the level of T6 aligned to the left of the spine. It was therefore decided that the UAC had been inadvertently inserted into the umbilical vein.

A blood gas sampled from the umbilical line showed: pH 7.55, pCO_2 2.5 kPa, pO_2 40 kPa

a. What are the most likely diagnoses?
    SELECT *TWO* ANSWERS ONLY
   i. Transposition of the great arteries
  ii. Eisenmenger's syndrome
 iii. Primary pulmonary hypertension
  iv. Right-sided aberrant subclavian artery
   v. Truncus arteriosus

b. What is the most appropriate investigation to confirm the diagnosis?
    SELECT *ONE* ANSWER ONLY
   i. Nitrogen wash-out test
  ii. Cardiac catheterisation
 iii. CT scan
  iv. Echocardiogram

ANSWERS TO CASE 6.14

a. i. Transposition of the great arteries
   iii. Primary pulmonary hypertension
b. iv. Echocardiogram

An AXR and a CXR are needed to check the course and position of an umbilical arterial catheter. In this case, it raised suspicion that a mere 12 cm "arterial catheter" can reach the level of T6 in a term average weight baby. An abdominal film would have demonstrated that the line did not go inferiorly to the iliac artery as an arterial catheter would. Transducing the umbilical line would also help distinguish an arterial and venous pressure trace.

These gas results show oxygenated blood from the UVC which is lying in the left atrium. However, the radial sample is deoxygenated blood suggesting cyanotic congenital heart disease. Differentials include transposition of the great arteries, pulmonary atresia, critical pulmonary stenosis (with PFO or VSD), total anomalous pulmonary venous congestion (obstructed type) and persistent fetal circulation (primary pulmonary hypertension).

CASE 6.15

A 6-year-old boy is admitted with a 5-day history of fever, lethargy, anorexia, jaundice and dark urine. On examination he is pyrexial, pale, mildly icteric with lymphadenopathy and tender hepatosplenomegaly. Initial investigations show:

Hb 5.5 g/dl
WCC 12.0 × 10⁹/l (N 41%, L 47%, M 11%, atypical lymphocytes 1%)
Platelets 212 × 10⁹/l
Bilirubin 37 μmol/l
Transaminases normal
Coagulation screen normal

a. What is the most likely diagnosis?
   SELECT THE *BEST* ANSWER
   i. Diamond–Blackfan anaemia
   ii. Sickle cell anaemia
   iii. Epstein–Barr infection
   iv. Hepatitis A
   v. Autoimmune haemolytic anaemia
   vi. Weil's disease

b. Which specific complications should be considered?
   SELECT *TWO* POSSIBLE ANSWERS
   i. Splenic haemorrhage
   ii. Severe haemolysis
   iii. Cerebral abscess
   iv. Cirrhosis
   v. Overwhelming sepsis

ANSWERS TO CASE 6.15

a. iii. Epstein–Barr infection
b. i. Splenic haemorrhage
    ii. Severe haemolysis

The most likely diagnosis is EBV infection (glandular fever/infectious mononucleosis) with associated acute haemolysis.

Complications include severe haemolysis and splenic haemorrhage. Neurological complications (e.g. seizures, ataxia, meningitis), airway obstruction (from tonsillar hypertrophy) and hepatitis are among other problems associated with EBV infections but were not apparent in this case.

Other investigations should include a monospot and EBV antibodies. An ultrasound scan should be performed to exclude splenic haemorrhage. Other causes of haemolysis should be considered especially if this boy is to be transfused.

An otherwise healthy 2-year-old boy is referred by his GP with a 2-day history of passing large dark, extremely offensive, non-mucousy stools. He has not had any diarrhoea or constipation, and there is no history of vomiting. He has recently complained of mild "tummy pain", but his appetite is unchanged and he has been able to sleep at night. On direct enquiry, there are no other symptoms of note. On examination, the youngster is pale and lethargic but alert. He is afebrile with a heart rate of 140 bpm, blood pressure of 85/30 mm Hg, and respiratory rate of 24 per min. The cardiovascular and respiratory systems are otherwise normal. He is tender periumbilically, but there is no organomegaly, palpable mass, rebound or guarding. Bowel sounds are reduced. The anal margin is normal.

Initial investigations reveal:

Hb 5.9 g/dl
CRP 6 g/l
WCC 10.2 × 10^9/l
albumin 36 g/l
platelets 158 × 10^9/l
Na 138 mmol/l
ESR 22 mm/h
K 4.9 mmol/l
PT 13 s
Urea 13.6 mmol/l
APTT 32 s
Creatinine 43 μmol/l
Fibrinogen 1.9 g/l

An AXR is unremarkable.

What is the most likely diagnosis?

SELECT *ONE* ANSWER ONLY
  i. Henoch–Schönlein purpura
  ii. Arteriovenous malformation
  iii. Von Willebrand's disease
  iv. Meckel's diverticulum
  v. Intussusception
  vi. Ulcerative colitis
  vii. Small bowel perforation

ANSWER TO CASE 6.16

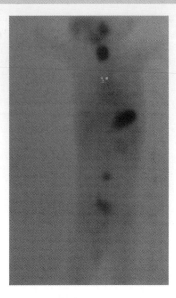

Fig 6.16

iv. Meckel's diverticulum

This story is consistent with a diagnosis of Meckel's diverticulum with ectopic gastric mucosa. This child presented with painless melaena, of which the most common cause at this age is bleeding associated with a Meckel's diverticulum. Intussusception is an important differential diagnosis. Melaena or partially altered blood in the absence of vomiting, significant abdominal pain, a palpable mass and with an unremarkable AXR collectively mediates against the diagnosis of intussusception in this case. Other rare causes of this presentation include upper gastrointestinal arteriovenous malformation and duodenal ulceration. Meckel's diverticulum occurs in 2% of all infants, symptoms usually presenting in the first 2 years of life. Acid secreted from ectopic mucosa lining the diverticulum causes ulceration of the normal adjacent ileal mucosa with consequent bleeding. A Meckel's diverticulum may act as a lead point for intussusception. Acute diverticulitis may mimic acute appendicitis.

Confirmation is made with technetium scintigraphy. In a "Meckel's scan" (see Fig. 6.16), technetium is taken up by the mucus-secreting cells of the ectopic gastric mucosa, facilitating visualisation of the diverticulum. The scan sensitivity is as high as 85% when uptake is enhanced by cimetidine or glucagon, and specificity is 95%. Surgical excision is curative.

A 12-year-old girl is referred by her GP with the "peculiar problem of marked muscle stiffness, pain, immobility and fatigue following exercise". She is otherwise quite well, has not been missing school and is described as a keen athlete. In retrospect, symptoms of post-exercise muscle fatigue date from the age of 6 years but have been worse over the past year. There is no similar family history and the physical examination proves to be normal.

a. What muscle disorder is the most likely cause?
   SELECT *ONE* ANSWER ONLY
   i. Myasthenia gravis
   ii. Myotonic dystrophy
   iii. Fascio-scapulo-humeral dystrophy
   iv. McArdle's disease
   v. Polymyalgia rheumatica
   vi. Fabry's disease

b. What further investigations would be relevant?
   SELECT *TWO* ANSWERS ONLY
   i. Anoxic exercise testing
   ii. Gene analysis
   iii. Tensilon test
   iv. Muscle biopsy
   v. Acute phase reactants
   vi. Creatinine kinase

ANSWERS TO CASE 6.17

a. iv. McArdle's disease
b. i. Anoxic exercise testing
    iv. Muscle biopsy

This girl has McArdle's disease. While several different disorders would need to be considered, the presentation of fatigue with anaerobic exercise is most typical of Type V (McArdle) and Type VII (Tarui) glycogenoses and possibly one of the lipid myopathies (carnitine palmityl transferase deficiency).

Investigations would include anoxic exercise testing using a blood pressure cuff, and measuring lactate pre- and post-exercise (a failure of the blood lactate to rise would be abnormal). A muscle biopsy would show increased glycogen and deficiency of specific enzymes.

There is no definitive management, but advice on general lifestyle and the avoidance of strenuous exercise would be important.

The prognosis is generally good, except for possible renal complications in adulthood associated with myoglobinuria.

CASE 6.18

A survey of 6000 singleton deliveries was undertaken to investigate the association between maternal smoking habits and the outcome of pregnancy. The following data were produced:

Table 6.18.1

	Perinatal deaths		Survivors		Births
Non-smokers	60	(a)	3940	(b)	4000
Ex-smokers	8	(c)	492	(d)	500
Smokers	39	(e)	1461	(f)	1500
Total	107		5893		6000

a. What is the overall perinatal mortality rate per 1000?
   SELECT *ONE* ANSWER ONLY
   i. 107/5893
   ii. 107/6000
   iii. 107/5893 × 1000
   iv. 107/6000 × 1000

b. What is the relative risk of perinatal death in the "smoking group" in comparison to the non-smoking group?
   SELECT *ONE* ANSWER ONLY

   i. $\dfrac{e/(e+f)}{a/(a+b)}$

   ii. $\dfrac{a/(e+f)}{f/(a+b)}$

   iii. $\dfrac{(e+f)/a}{(a+b)/e}$

   iv. $\dfrac{(e+f)/e}{(a+b)/a}$

c. What statistical test could you use on this data to strengthen your conclusion?
   SELECT THE *BEST* ANSWER
   i. Paired t-test
   ii. Chi-square
   iii. Regression analysis
   iv. Pearson correlation
   v. Non-parametric regression

ANSWERS TO CASE 6.18

a. iv. $107/6000 \times 1000$

b. i. $\dfrac{e/(e+f)}{a/(a+b)} = 1.73$

c. ii. Chi-square

Mortality rate for deaths that occur close to birth is usually calculated by:

$$\frac{\text{No. of deaths}}{\text{Total births}} \times 1000$$

The relative risk of perinatal death in the "smoking" group in comparison to the "non-smoking" group is calculated by:

$$\frac{\text{Perinatal mortality rate in the smoking group}}{\text{Perinatal mortality rate in the non-smoking group}} = \frac{39/1000}{60/4000} = 1.73$$

The confidence interval is calculated from the relative risk. The 95% CI for this relative risk is 1.16–2.58. When interpreting the CI, we look to see if it contains 1, as this is the value of the relative risk that would indicate that there was no statistically significant difference between the risk in smoking mothers and non-smoking mothers. This CI only contains values greater than 1, with the possibility of a relative risk as high as 2.58. However, it is important not to over interpret this CI as the lower limit is very close to 1. In order to strengthen your conclusion, it would be useful to derive a p value for the null hypothesis; there is no difference in the risk of perinatal death between mothers that smoke and mothers that don't smoke. An estimate for the p value can be obtained by performing a Chi-square test on the data. The formula for obtaining the Chi-square statistic is:

$$\chi^2 = \sum \frac{(\text{observed} - \text{expected})^2}{\text{expected}}$$

This statistic measures the discrepancy between the observed counts in the table and the counts you would expect under the null hypothesis. For example, there were 99 deaths in total so if there were no differences between smoking and non-smoking mothers, the expected number of perinatal deaths to mothers that didn't smoke would be:

$$99 \times = \frac{4000}{5500} = 72$$

The following 2×2 table illustrates the observed and expected values

Table 6.18.2

	Died		Survived		
	Observed	Expected	Observed	Expected	Total births
Mother didn't smoke	60	72	3940	3928	4000
Mother smoked	39	27	1461	1473	1500
Total	99		5401		5500

The figures in the above table are then entered into the formula for the Chi-square statistic illustrated above. With reference to a table of Chi-square values, the calculated value is greater than the tabulated value at a significance level of 1%, indicating $p = <0.01$. Thus we have evidence to suggest that the null hypothesis should be rejected.

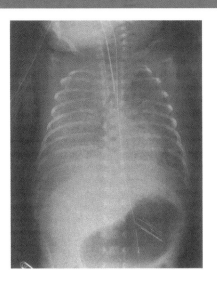

Fig 6.19

A 35-year-old Irish woman with polyhydramnios was delivered vaginally of a female infant at 32 weeks' gestation. The antenatal ultrasound had shown a large abdominal cyst. Intubation was performed electively on the neonatal unit. The AXR is shown.

What are the findings on the X-ray?

SELECT *TWO* ANSWERS ONLY
  i. Oesophageal atresia
 ii. Pulmonary hypoplasia
iii. Bowel perforation
 iv. Hepatomegaly
  v. Calcified abdominal mass
 vi. Cardiomegaly
vii. Thoracic compression

ANSWERS TO CASE 6.19

v. Calcified abdominal mass

vii. Thoracic compression

The X-ray shows a large abdominal calcified cyst with compression of the thoracic structures.

Possible diagnoses include an ovarian cyst, choledochal cyst, mesenteric cyst, omental cyst, enteric duplication, meconium pseudocyst or cystic teratoma.

It is important here to exclude cystic fibrosis.

Investigations that would be relevant include a postnatal ultrasound, DNA analysis for CF mutations, and cyst histology at laparotomy.

Outcome

The lesion was a meconium pseudocyst, calcification of the cyst suggesting the diagnosis of a meconium pseudocyst or a cystic teratoma. Laparotomy identified a segment of adherent bowel containing a perforation with resultant inflammation, fibrosis and calcification. The mucosal gland pattern was not consistent with cystic fibrosis. DNA analysis excluded the 20 common mutations in the Northern Ireland population and there was no family history of CF. This antenatal diagnosis may be associated with cystic fibrosis but can also occur in other diagnoses, e.g. volvulus or ileal atresia.

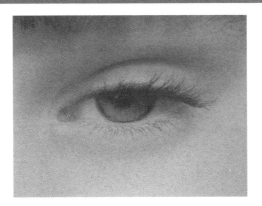

Fig 6.20

The 4-year-old daughter of a pharmacist was referred by her optician with reduced visual acuity and bilateral red eyes. Between referral and review, she developed swelling of her left ankle and knee, and stiffness in her neck. On examination, the swollen joints were all warm with mild limitation of movement but no fixed flexion deformity. Remaining examination was unremarkable except for her eyes, which showed keratic precipitates as a complication of anterior uveitis.

What is the most likely underlying diagnosis?

SELECT *ONE* ANSWER ONLY
  i. Rheumatoid arthritis
 ii. Systemic lupus erythematosus
iii. Systemic sclerosis
 iv. Reiter's disease
  v. Still's disease
 vi. Type I pauciarticular JIA

ANSWER TO CASE 6.20

vi. Type I pauciarticular JIA

Keratic precipitates are seen as fine white lines visible over the central cornea. They consist of inflammatory cells from iris and uveal vessels which stick to the corneal endothelium. Anterior uveitis is found in a number of inflammatory, auto-immune and infectious diseases. It may be unilateral or bilateral. Early changes may be subtle and detectable only by slit lamp examination. Management concentrates on determining a systemic aetiology, preserving visual function, reducing ocular pain and eliminating inflammation. Anterior uveitis is seen in 15-30% of patients with pauciarticular JIA. Joint involvement may be mild or not evident at the time of ophthalmic diagnosis. The severity of the joint disease does not correlate with the risk of eye involvement. For this reason, all children with a diagnosis of pauciarticular JIA need 3-monthly slit lamp examinations for at least the first 5 years of disease. Ninety per cent of patients have positive antinuclear antibodies. Neither rheumatoid factor nor HLAB27 is associated. In type I pauciarticular JIA, joint disease normally occurs before the fourth birthday. Type I is more common in girls who are at greater risk of chronic anterior uveitis (iridocyclitis). Type II primarily affects older boys who may subsequently develop spondyloarthropathy.

Ophthalmological complications of anterior uveitis include posterior synechiae, acute glaucoma, cataracts, phthisis bulbi (degeneration of the globe) and permanent blindness. Posterior synechiae refers to adherence of the iris to the anterior lens capsule. Caught early, it can be treated with cycloplegics. Progressive disease leads to glaucoma and requires surgical management. Cataracts may form as a result of chronic inflammation or secondary to long-term topical or systemic steroid use. Phthisis bulbi is atrophy of the globe; this is managed by enucleation for cosmetic reasons. Finally, in the absence of globe degeneration, permanent blindness may result.

Chapter 7

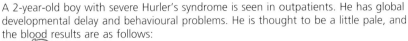

CASE 7.1

A 2-year-old boy with severe Hurler's syndrome is seen in outpatients. He has global developmental delay and behavioural problems. He is thought to be a little pale, and the blood results are as follows:

Hb 3.9 g/dl
MCV 54 fl
WCC 4.1 × 10^9/l
platelets 206 × 10^9/l

a. What is the most likely diagnosis?
   SELECT ONE ANSWER ONLY
   i. G6PD deficiency
   ii. Acute lymphoblastic leukaemia
   iii. Fanconi anaemia
   iv. Severe iron deficiency anaemia
   v. Meckel's diverticulum

b. What treatment is required?
   SELECT ONE ANSWER ONLY
   i. Irradiated packed cells
   ii. Intravenous iron sucrose
   iii. Oral iron supplementation
   iv. Dietetic advice
   v. Bone marrow transplant
   vi. Blood transfusion

ANSWERS TO CASE 7.1

a. iv. Severe iron deficiency
b. iii. Oral iron supplementation

Hurler's syndrome is type I mucopolysaccharidosis. Although normal at birth, dysmorphic features develop after the first year of life. Developmental regression is usually severe. In this patient, the developmental delay and behavioural problems meant that he ate very poorly. His dietary intake of iron was virtually nil and anaemia developed chronically.

As the patient is not compromised by the anaemia, immediate blood transfusion is unnecessary, and may even be dangerous. Iron supplementation will have an effect in 2-3 days.

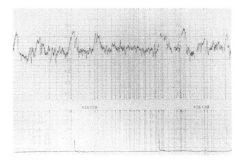

Fig 7.2

At 38 weeks' gestation a 25-year-old woman presented with reduced fetal movements and therefore had a cardiotocograph performed.

a. Identify three main features (normal or abnormal) of the fetal heart rate on the CTG?
SELECT THE *THREE* BEST ANSWERS
  i. Fetal tachycardia
  ii. Normal baseline fetal heart rate
  iii. Hyperreactive trace
  iv. Reactive trace
  v. Type I decelerations
  vi. Type II accelerations
  vii. Normal beat-to-beat variation

b. In the presence of an abnormal trace, which of the following is not a risk factor for the development of fetal hypoxia and acidosis?
SELECT THE *BEST* ANSWER
  i. Intrauterine growth restriction
  ii. Infant of a diabetic mother
  iii. Reversed end diastolic flow
  iv. Intrauterine infection
  v. Prematurity
  vi. Post term

ANSWERS TO CASE 7.2

a. ii. Normal baseline fetal heart rate
    iv. Reactive trace
    vii. Normal beat-to-beat variation
b. ii. Infant of a diabetic mother

The normal baseline fetal heart rate is between 110 and 150 bpm.

Normal baseline variability is between 10 and 25 bpm.

This CTG is reactive: it shows normal variability around a normal baseline, with normal accelerations of the fetal heart rate (due to fetal movements or uterine contractions).

There are no decelerations; the fetal heart rate does not fall below 110 bpm throughout the trace.

Risk factors for hypoxia and acidosis include: intra-uterine growth restriction, intra-uterine infection, prematurity, post term (>41 weeks' gestation), placental abruption, and placental insufficiency.

Different delivery units may have slightly different guidelines but generally a paediatrician needs to be present for the following deliveries: prematurity (<36 weeks' gestation), small for gestational age, fetal distress (thick meconium stained liquor, abnormal trace, fetal scalp pH <7.20), multiple pregnancy, significant antepartum haemorrhage, fetal disease (congenital abnormality, rhesus disease).

A10-day-old boy was referred for endocrine evaluation due to persistent jaundice, episodes of hypoglycaemia, difficulty with temperature regulation and small genitalia. He was born at term by forceps delivery and required bag and mask resuscitation. His Apgar scores were 3 at 1 min, 7 at 5 min and 8 at 10 min. He was admitted to the neonatal unit for i.v. glucose and settled before being transferred to the postnatal ward. Septic screen was negative. On examination, he was jaundiced, had no obvious dysmorphic features and had a small penis with hypoplastic scrotum. Both testes were felt in the scrotum. In view of his persistent symptoms, he had the following investigations:

Blood group A+ve
Mother's blood group A +ve
Direct Coomb's test negative
TSH 1.7 mU/l (normal range 0.5-6 mU/l)
Thyroxine 57 nmol/l (normal range 90-220 nmol/l)
Cortisol 41.3 nmol/l (normal range 180-700 nmol/l)

The result of a glucagon stimulation test was as follows:

Table 7.3.1

Time (min)	−15	0	30	60	90	120	150	180
Glucose (mmol/l)	3.9	3.7	4.0	4.3	4.0	3.3	4.7	3.0
GH (mU/l)	3.7	3.8	3.8	6.0	9.7	9.4	6.9	6.9
Cortisol (nmol/l)	<70				<70		<70	<70

Glucose was administered i.v. at 120 min, as the bedside BM was 1.6 mmol/l.

Other baseline endocrine tests showed:
FSH <1 IU/l
LH <0.3 IU/l
Testosterone 1.9 nmol/l
ACTH <10 ng/l

The urinary steroid profile showed that steroid levels were fairly low suggestive of some degree of hypoadrenal hypofunction.

What is the likely diagnosis?

SELECT *ONE* ANSWER ONLY
i. Hyperinsulinism
ii. Congenital adrenal hyperplasia
iii. Congenital hypothyroidism
iv. Congenital hypopituitarism
v. Congenital adrenal hypoplasia
vi. Conn's syndrome

ANSWER TO CASE 7.3

iv. Congenital hypopituitarism

Congenital hypopituitarism (CH) is the likely diagnosis. Mutations in the pituitary developmental transcription factor genes (POU1F1, PROP1 or HESX1) account for the majority of cases of CH. Dynamic pituitary testing shows a very inadequate cortisol and GH response in a neonate. The combination of GH and ACTH deficiencies in the newborn may result in severe hypoglycaemia that responds only to hormone replacement. Prolonged jaundice in a neonate should prompt the measurement of thyroid function. Thyroid function shows low levels of T4 with normal TSH, confirming pituitary hypothyroidism. The combination of small penis and hypoplastic scrotum suggests hypogonadotrophic hypogonadism but LH and FSH levels are difficult to interpret in the immediate neonatal period.

An MRI of the hypothalamic pituitary area is needed to help confirm the diagnosis. In approximately half of all patients with CH, there is attenuation or interruption of the pituitary stalk with or without associated corpus callosum defects. Risk of intellectual disability is higher if the patient has a defect in corpus callosum. In this case, there was a hold-up of the neurosecretory granules at the level of the hypothalamus. Ophthalmological assessment should be performed to look for optic nerve atrophy. Measurement of gonadotrophins at about 3 months may help to confirm hypogonadotrophic hypogonadism as there is a natural surge in the hormones in the first few months of life.

Management involves the instigation of a replacement dose of hydrocortisone (8–10 mg/m²) and thyroxine (100 mcg/m²). In this case, resolution of hypoglycaemia occurred, but sometimes GH replacement in addition may be necessary at this early stage. The parents need to be given appropriate information as to the dose adjustment of hydrocortisone during intercurrent illnesses (i.e. doubling of dose of hydrocortisone) and taught how to use i.m. hydrocortisone in case of emergency. Assuming the hypoglycaemia resolves with hydrocortisone, consideration for GH replacement can be deferred initially. Puberty will need to be induced at 12 years (assuming no spontaneous puberty) with testosterone.

A 9-year-old girl presented with a large swelling in her neck which had been increasing in size for 2 weeks. She had been feeling unwell with a slight temperature. On examination there was a 4 cm × 3 cm swelling anterior to the left sternomastoid which was erythematous and mildly tender; it became fluctuant over the next few days. Serology to *Bartonella henselae* was positive.

Investigations showed:
    Hb 12.6 g/dl
    WCC 8.6 × 10^9/l
    Platelets 355 × 10^9/l
    CRP 12 mg/l

a. What is the diagnosis?
    SELECT *ONE* ANSWER ONLY
  i. Atypical mycobacterial infection
 ii. Cat-scratch disease
iii. Lyme disease
 iv. Lymphogranuloma venereum
  v. Wegener's granulomatosis

b. What complications of this disease may occur?
    SELECT *TWO* POSSIBLE ANSWERS
  i. Cardiomyopathy
 ii. Myelitis
iii. Encephalopathy
 iv. Glomerulonephritis
  v. Thrombocytosis
 vi. Peripheral neuropathy

ANSWERS TO CASE 7.4

a. ii. Cat-scratch disease
b. ii. Myelitis
   iii. Encephalopathy

It is important to elicit whether there is a history suggesting recent infection in the head or neck, e.g. sore throat, scalp infection, etc.; if there has been any contact with tuberculosis or unpasteurised milk? Any contact with cats? Or any foreign travel?

Investigations should include: FBC and film; viral serology, including EBV and CMV, and serology to *Bartonella henselae*, which causes cat-scratch disease; CXR and Mantoux, to help differentiate from TB; and biopsy of the swelling may be considered.

In 75% of cases of cat–scratch disease, a lesion appears at the site of inoculation between 3 and 10 days after the scratch. The commonest site of lymphadenopathy is the axilla.

In uncomplicated cases, no treatment is required. Typically the swelling slowly resolves, unless there is an underlying immunodeficiency. If treatment is needed, rifampicin, cotrimoxazole, ciprofloxacin or gentamicin can be used.

Numerous complications have been reported, the most common being neurological, including encephalopathy, cranial and peripheral nerve lesions and myelitis. Hepatitis, osteomyelitis and thrombocytopenia purpura can also occur.

CASE 7.5

A 6-week-old breast-fed baby boy is referred to a paediatrician because he is failing to thrive. He was born at term with a birth weight of 3900 g and no perinatal problems. Since 2 weeks of age, he has been described as chesty and this was felt to be due to an upper respiratory tract infection, as his older brother was suffering from one at the time. Four weeks later and after a course of antibiotics, he is no better and is now appearing pale and sweaty when feeding.

On examination, he appears thin, his weight being on the 10th centile. There are no signs of intercurrent viral illness. Although not overly distressed, he is tachypnoeic and has intercostal recession. His oxygen saturation is 82% in air. He is tachycardic. His pulses are rather weak. There is a right parasternal heave and a systolic murmur heard at the pulmonary area with a widely split second sound and a loud P2. ECG indicates right atrial and ventricular enlargement. CXR shows a large heart, increased pulmonary vascularity and a large square shaped supracardiac shadow.

a. What is the likely diagnosis?
SELECT *ONE* ANSWER ONLY
   i. Patent ductus arteriosus
  ii. Truncus arteriosus
 iii. Total anomalous pulmonary venous drainage
  iv. Transposition of the great vessels
   v. Large VSD

b. What treatment is initially indicated?
SELECT *ONE* ANSWER ONLY
   i. Indomethacin
  ii. Diuretics
 iii. Prostaglandin infusion
  iv. Urgent cardiac surgical opinion
   v. ACE inhibitors

ANSWERS TO CASE 7.5

a. iii. Total anomalous pulmonary venous drainage
b. iv. Urgent cardiac surgical opinion

The diagnosis is unobstructed total anomalous pulmonary venous drainage. In this infant, the pulmonary veins formed a confluence which drained into the superior vena cava causing total common mixing and marked volume overloading of the right heart. The child was therefore mildly cyanosed and breathless. In this infant, blood was able to reach the left side of the heart through a large ASD. In some children with an intact atrial septum or restrictive ASD, there may be a significant hypoplasia of the left side of the heart. There are three types of total anomalous pulmonary venous drainage – supracardiac, as in this case, cardiac or infracardiac. The lesion can also be obstructed or non–obstructed. Obstructed cases tend to present with severe respiratory distress and cyanosis in the neonatal period, the severe pulmonary venous congestion on X–ray often leading to a misdiagnosis as respiratory disease. If pulmonary venous return is obstructed, however, the radiological clue is marked pulmonary venous congestion and hepatomegaly with a *small* heart shadow.

The condition is a paediatric cardiac surgical emergency and therefore the child should have an urgent echocardiogram and be transferred to a paediatric cardiac unit as soon as possible. For those children who survive to surgery, there is around a 10% early mortality. Thereafter the prognosis is best for those children who do not have pulmonary arterial hypertension.

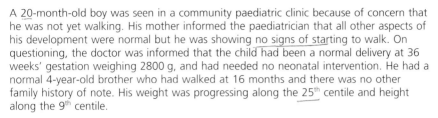
CASE 7.6

A 20-month-old boy was seen in a community paediatric clinic because of concern that he was not yet walking. His mother informed the paediatrician that all other aspects of his development were normal but he was showing no signs of starting to walk. On questioning, the doctor was informed that the child had been a normal delivery at 36 weeks' gestation weighing 2800 g, and had needed no neonatal intervention. He had a normal 4-year-old brother who had walked at 16 months and there was no other family history of note. His weight was progressing along the 25th centile and height along the 9th centile.

What is the most likely diagnosis in this case?

SELECT *ONE* ANSWER ONLY

  i. Global developmental delay with late walking
 ii. Mild cerebral palsy
iii. Becker muscular dystrophy
 iv. Duchenne muscular dystrophy
  v. Normal variant
 vi. Myasthenia gravis

ANSWER TO CASE 7.6

v. Normal variant

A detailed assessment of all aspects of development is needed:
- speech – he should have approximately 5 words and may be using simple combinations
- social – manages a cup/demands objects by pointing
- fine motor – scribbles/turns 2-3 book pages at a time/builds tower of three blocks
- gross motor – pulling to stand/cruising

Are there any specific features such as crawling or bottom shuffling or demonstration of a Gower's manoeuvre?

A thorough physical examination including neurodevelopmental assessment is required.

The diagnoses to be considered fall into two main groups:
1. Normal variant late walkers:
   These will develop normally. Indications of this are rolling, creeping or bottom shuffling. Other features may be reduced tone especially of the lower limbs, late sitting, lax joints and a family history of late walking. Ninety-seven per cent of children walk by 18 months of age (6 steps unaided).
2. Newly diagnosed conditions which may present with late walking:
   a. Duchenne muscular dystrophy – affects 1 : 3500 males and is diagnosed by elevated CPK and muscle biopsy
   b. Cerebral palsy – mild or moderate spastic diplegia may present as late walking
   c. Learning difficulties – late walking may be the first sign of global delay

This child was a normal variant late walker who started to walk 2 weeks later.

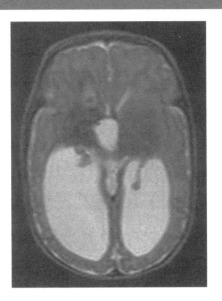

Fig 7.7

A preterm infant was born at 25 weeks' gestation. The cranial ultrasound scan taken on day 1 of life was normal. On day 2, the infant suffered a profound collapse and required resuscitation. Figure 7.7 shows a T2-weighted MRI brain scan taken at 13 weeks' postnatal age.

What is the most likely diagnosis?

SELECT *ONE* ANSWER ONLY

  i. Hydrancephaly
 ii. Bilateral subdural haemorrhages
iii. Parenchymal leukomalacia
 iv. Post-haemorrhagic ventricular dilatation
  v. Cerebral atrophy

ANSWER TO CASE 7.7

iv. Post-haemorrhagic ventricular dilatation

Acute clinical consequences of a large intraventricular haemorrhage include acidaemia, hypotension, seizures, anaemia and impaired consciousness.

The infant's head circumference increased by two centile lines between 38 and 40 weeks corrected gestational age. He was irritable, feeding poorly and vomiting occasionally. A ventricular tap was performed.

The next step in management would be to refer the baby for a neurosurgical opinion. The infant may require a ventricular reservoir device to enable frequent CSF aspiration to be carried out more safely. The infant may ultimately require a ventricular shunt.

Procedure: ventricular tap

The surface landmark used for the ventricular tap is the lateral margin of the anterior fontanelle, not medial to the pupillary line. A medial passage could result in aspiration of the dural sinus. The needle should be directed forwards and slightly inwards towards the inner canthus of the opposite eye. Insertion should not exceed 4-5 cm and will often aspirate CSF at a shallow depth of 1 cm in infants with post-haemorrhagic ventricular dilatation.

CASE 7.8

A 22-month-old girl presented with a 7-day history of upper respiratory symptoms and 2 days of swollen legs. She was not eating well and occasionally complained of abdominal pains but remained active. She was a full-term normal delivery with no past medical history of note. She was not on any medication and the rest of the family was well. On examination she was well but had markedly oedematous legs. Her blood pressure was 125/85 and pulse 120/min. She had a distended abdomen with shifting dullness. Investigations: Hb 13.4 g/dl, WCC 15.0×10^9/l, platelets 676×10^9/l, Na 138 mmol/l, K 4.3 mmol/l, urea 4.5 mmol/l, and creatinine 32 μmol/l.

a. What two other investigations would you request?
   SELECT *TWO* ANSWERS ONLY
   i. Abdominal ultrasound
   ii. Pulse oximetry
   iii. Urinalysis
   iv. Blood protein
   v. Serum osmolality
   vi. Four-limb blood pressure

b. What other blood result is likely to be abnormally high in this condition?
   SELECT *ONE* ANSWER ONLY
   i. IgA
   ii. Coagulation inhibitors
   iii. C3
   iv. Lipids

c. What would your management be?
   SELECT *TWO* ANSWERS ONLY
   i. Fluid restriction
   ii. High protein diet
   iii. Steroids
   iv. i.v. albumin infusion
   v. i.v. immunoglobulin

ANSWERS TO CASE 7.8

a. iii. Urinalysis
   iv. Blood protein
b. iv. Lipids
c. i. Fluid restriction
   iii. Steroids

This child has nephrotic syndrome. Nephrotic syndrome is characterised by massive urinary protein loss leading to hypoproteinaemia and oedema. The cause of the protein loss is unknown but capillary membrane permeability is increased. This increased filtered load overcomes the tubular reabsorption capacity, hence proteinuria. The plasma oncotic pressure falls and causes oedema. With progression of the disease the intravascular volume becomes depleted and the renin-angiotensin system is stimulated. This may lead to hypertension.

The liver increases protein synthesis in order to try to maintain adequate plasma albumin levels. As a consequence, plasma lipoprotein levels increase. However, lower levels of plasma lipoprotein lipase are also present and both factors lead to raised plasma cholesterol and lipids.

Of all childhood nephrotic syndrome, 90% is idiopathic; of these, 85% is minimal change nephrosis on histopathology; 5% have mesangio-proliferative type and 10% focal glomerular sclerosis; the remainder is congenital or associated with glomerulonephritis, tumours or drugs.

The most frequent complication of nephrotic syndrome is infection. There are many theories for why this is so, such as loss of immunoglobulins and complement proteins in the urine. *Streptococcus pneumoniae* is the most common pathogen and penicillin prophylaxis is therefore recommended. There is also an increased incidence of thrombosis, both venous and arterial.

Treatment consists of fluid if there is any evidence of intravascular volume depletion, then fluid restriction, accurate fluid intake and output measurements, daily weights, and continuing urinalysis and steroids. Most cases are responsive to steroid therapy. If there is no response after one month, renal biopsy is indicated. Relapses are treated in the same way as the initial episode. Frequent relapsers may need a long course of steroids or other drugs, e.g. cyclophosphamide, to put them into remission. In most children, steroid responsive nephritic syndrome will have resolved by the end of the second decade.

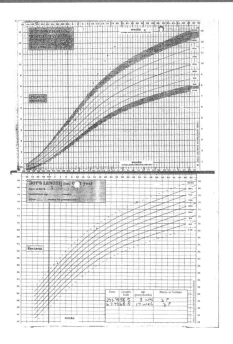

Fig 7.9

A 5-month-old boy was referred by his GP to paediatric outpatients because his weight was "escalating off the top of his growth chart with no signs of reaching a plateau". His development was normal. His growth chart is shown.

a. Which pieces of information would help you make a diagnosis?
   SELECT *THREE* ANSWERS ONLY
   i. Neonatal history of overfeeding
   ii. Maternal drug history in pregnancy
   iii. History of floppiness
   iv. History of hypoglycaemia
   v. Sleeping pattern
   vi. History of diarrhoea
   vii. Head circumference

b. Which of the following diagnoses would be most likely?
   SELECT *ONE* ANSWER ONLY
   i. Laurence-Moon-Biedl syndrome
   ii. Overfeeding
   iii. Prader–Willi syndrome
   iv. Congenital hypothyroidism
   v. Zellweger syndrome
   vi. Rubenstein–Taybi
   vii. Diabetes mellitus

ANSWERS TO CASE 7.9

a. iii. History of floppiness
 iv. History of hypoglycaemia
 vii. Head circumference
b. ii. Overfeeding

In the first year of life, growth is almost entirely nutrition-dependent. By the age of 2 years, GH receptors are present, and hormonal causes become significant.

It is important to elicit a thorough dietary history of any child referred for growth concerns. This includes what the feeds consist of, how formula feeds are made up, and how much and how often feeds are given. A developmental history would help distinguish certain syndromes such as Soto's and Prader–Willi. Children with Prader–Willi are characteristically small and hypotonic at birth, with a history of poor feeding. The size of other family members and the child's head circumference should also be measured.

Rare causes that should be considered:

Soto's syndrome (cerebral gigantism) – characteristics include a large child, commonly with developmental delay.

Beckwith–Wiedemann – characteristics include obesity, hyperinsulinaemic hypoglycaemia, macroglossia, exomphalos, visceromegaly, and parallel creases on the ear lobes.

Prader–Willi – characteristics include obesity, developmental delay, hypotonia, short stature, hypogonadism and diabetes mellitus. These children are characteristically small at birth, with a history of poor feeding; typically, obesity occurs after the first year.

Laurence–Moon–Biedl – characteristics include short stature, hypogonadism, diabetes insipidus, polydactyly and retinitis pigmentosa. Obesity characteristically occurs after the first year.

A 15-week-old infant was admitted to the paediatric ward with a history of possible choking. Her mother reported that she had noted a mild cough at lunchtime that had settled quickly and she had thought no more about it. However, that evening whilst in the bath the infant had begun coughing again, this time more violently. Despite there being no apparent history of foreign body aspiration her mother still described the episode as a choking type cough. The baby had not fed for 4 hours previously. The GP was called and felt the air entry to be markedly different on each side and queried a pneumothorax. The baby had previously been well.

On arrival she was pink and well perfused. She fed well and was happy and smiling. Oxygen saturations were 96% in room air. She was afebrile with some peri-nasal crusting and had mild to moderate sternal recession. Air entry was decreased over the left lung. However, on review by the registrar, when she was asleep, there was minimal respiratory distress and air entry was said to be normal. A diagnosis of upper respiratory tract infection was felt to be more likely.

The following morning she was reviewed. Again she had moderate sternal recession and markedly decreased air entry over the left lung.

a. What are the possible diagnoses?
   SELECT *TWO* ANSWERS ONLY
   i. Bronchiolitis
   ii. Foreign body
   iii. Mural or extra-mural obstruction of the left main bronchus
   iv. Gastro-oesophageal reflux with aspiration
   v. Cystic fibrosis

b. Choose the most appropriate initial investigations?
   SELECT *TWO* ANSWERS ONLY
   i. Bronchoscopy
   ii. CXR
   iii. Sweat test
   iv. Upper GI contrast
   v. pH study

ANSWERS TO CASE 7.10

a. ii. Foreign body
    iii. Mural or extra-mural obstruction of the left main bronchus
b. i. Bronchoscopy
    ii. CXR

A CXR was performed which, although rotated, suggested hyperluceny of the left lung. A CT scan of her chest suggested the diagnosis of bronchogenic cyst that was partially obstructing the left main bronchus. This was confirmed at thoracotomy where it was successfully removed. She subsequently made a good post-operative recovery.

A 2-day-old infant was admitted to the neonatal unit because a bluish discolouration was noted periorally, on the forehead and on both hands. Six hours later, his oxygen requirement gradually increased and he required 60% oxygen to maintain saturations around 93%. The following investigations were performed: CXR showed a normal cardiac shadow and clear lung fields; ECG was within normal limits; four-limb blood pressures were within normal limits; echocardiogram was normal; hyperoxia test was normal; and arterial blood gas in 40% oxygen was – pH 7.31, pCO2 6.1 kPa, pO2 18.12 kPa, BE −4.1.

What is the most likely diagnosis?

SELECT *ONE* ANSWER ONLY

  i. Persistent pulmonary hypertension of the newborn
 ii. Group B Strep septicaemia
iii. Methaemoglobinaemia
 iv. Cyanotic congenital heart disease
  v. Hyaline membrane disease

ANSWER TO CASE 7.11

iii. Methaemoglobinaemia

This infant has methaemoglobinaemia. A methaemoglobin level should be checked (normal <1%). A detailed family history and maternal drug history including the anaesthetic drugs given during delivery must be sought.

In normality, the oxidation of the iron moiety of haemoglobin from the ferrous to the ferric state results in the formation of methaemoglobin. Methaemoglobinaemia occurs when ferric haemoglobin cannot be converted back to ferrous haemoglobin by the normal reducing mechanisms. High concentrations of methaemoglobin lead to a reduced oxygen carrying capacity due to the red cells delivering less oxygen, and a left shift of the haemoglobin dissociation curve. Therefore, there is a reduction in the oxygen-carrying capacity of the red blood cell.

Methaemoglobinaemia may be congenital or acquired. The congenital form may be a familial autosomal recessive NADPH-cytochrome b5 reductase (diaphorase 1) deficiency or an autosomal dominant haemoglobin M disease. A number of substances are capable of oxidising haemoglobin directly and will do so in vitro; these include nitrites, nitrates, chlorates and quinines. The diagnosis in this case is autosomal recessive congenital methaemoglobinaemia.

CASE 7.12

A 2-year-old Caucasian girl, unwell with a 24 h history of fever and vomiting was referred by her GP who noted that she had a maculo-papular "flea-bitten" rash on her trunk. Her mother reports that the child had become worse in the last hour, the rash had spread to her limbs, and she now appeared confused. On examination she was tachycardic (pulse 140 bpm) with a capillary refill time of 4 s and had no meningism. Some of the maculo-papular lesions were now 3-4 mm large and non-blanching.

Which diagnosis should be considered as a matter of priority?

SELECT *ONE* ANSWER ONLY

   i. Rocky Mountain Spotted fever
  ii. Acute lymphoblastic leukaemia
 iii. Meningococcal septicaemia
 iv. Bleeding diathesis
   v. Henoch–Schonlein Purpura
 vi. Lyme disease
vii. Necrotizing fasciitis

ANSWER TO CASE 7.12

iii. Meningococcal septicaemia

Meningococcal septicaemia is the most important diagnosis to consider, and a maculo-papular "flea-bitten" rash may precede the typical purpuric rash in many children. This fulminant presentation is typical of meningococcaemia, but haemorrhagic rashes may also be caused by Henoch–Schonlein Purpura (HSP), acute lymphoblastic leukaemia, bleeding diatheses, and in travellers returning from North America, Rocky Mountain spotted fever.

The immediate management is critical in reducing mortality, and early consideration of the diagnosis is important. Management should be proactive, anticipating problems rather than responding to them. Elicit senior clinical support, with sufficient hands to stabilise and manage the child rapidly. Establish venous access (at two sites), and give a fluid bolus of 20 mg/kg normal saline or colloid, and an i.v. beta lactam antibiotic (e.g. cefotaxime/ceftriaxone). Assess the response and repeat if necessary. Consider an inotrope infusion, and if more than 40 ml/kg of fluid has been required to stabilise, it is advisable to intubate and ventilate early. Local policy will determine whether one transfers the child when stable to PICU or to a regional referral unit.

Blood should be taken for FBC and differential count, clotting studies, U&E, and, depending on severity, blood gases. Pulse, respiratory rate, blood pressure and core and peripheral temperatures should be monitored. Blood cultures are usually positive in children who have not received prior antibiotics, and Gram staining of an impression slide from a skin scraping of a purpuric lesion can give an immediate result, even following antibiotics. PCR results are now available in less than a week in the UK (use an EDTA tube). Serology may be helpful, but requires both acute and convalescent samples.

The GP should give parenteral penicillin prior to referral, if diagnosis is considered. Public Health usually arranges antibiotic chemo-prophylaxis for close contacts, usually rifampicin 10 mg/kg (maximum 600 mg) b.d. for 2 days. Alternatives are a single i.m. dose of ceftriaxone, or oral ciprofloxacin. Public Health will also be aware of possible clusters of disease, which may require wider antibiotic chemoprophylaxis, and for group C disease – immunization. They can also alert the community to recognise and report symptoms and signs early.

Meningococcal C conjugate vaccine is now given in the routine immunisation schedule in the UK, and has dramatically reduced the prevalence of disease. There is also a polysaccharide vaccine for groups A, C, W135 and Y, but not for the commonest UK group B. Antibiotic chemo-prophylaxis, given early to close contacts reduces secondary cases.

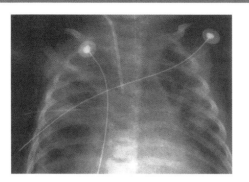

Fig 7.13

A 6-year-old boy with no past medical history of note has this chest radiograph during the recovery phase after a recent severe pneumonic illness.

What are these appearances likely to be due to?

SELECT *ONE* ANSWER ONLY
   i. Pneumocystis carinii
  ii. Right-sided diaphragmatic hernia
 iii. Congenital cystic adenomatoid malformation of the lung
  iv. Pneumatocoeles
   v. Clostridial infection
  vi. Hydatid disease

ANSWER TO CASE 7.13

iv. Pneumatocoeles

The chest X-ray demonstrates that the patient is intubated with the tip of the endotracheal tube in a satisfactory position. A right internal jugular venous line is also present with the tip probably in the superior vena cava. Cardiac monitoring leads are also noted, as is the presence of a nasogastric tube and chest drain. These lines and tubes indicate that the pneumonia was quite severe. Within the lungs are bilateral multiple ring shadows which are relatively symmetrical, measuring up to 4-5 cm in diameter. The thickness of their walls is quite regular and thin. Air-fluid levels are not seen within them. All areas of the lungs are affected. There is probably a small residual pneumothorax at the right costophrenic angle and right-sided subcutaneous surgical emphysema.

The most likely cause of multiple cystic air collections in the lungs following pneumonia is the development of pneumatocoeles. These are interstitial accumulations of air probably due to obstructive over-inflation. They are characteristically seen following bacterial pneumonia, particularly due to Staphylococcus aureus (the diagnosis in this case), but also from other bacteria, including H. influenzae, streptococcus, klebsiella, E. coli, and M. tuberculosis. They may rapidly enlarge and cause mediastinal displacement and even perforate into the pleural space causing a pyopneumothorax. In a patient with pneumonia, they can, on occasion, be difficult to differentiate from a lung abscess, and in fact there is no foolproof method for radiologically making such a differentiation, particularly if inflammatory exudate from a surrounding infected area seeps into them and gives rise to an air-fluid level. Pneumatocoeles are more commonly multiple than lung abscesses and more often have a thin smooth wall. In addition, clinical differentiation should be possible since pneumatocoeles usually develop during the healing phase (10-14 days into the course of the infection) while the patient is clinically improving whereas a lung abscess develops early on, while the patient is still quite ill. Other causes of similar pneumatocoeles include hydrocarbon aspiration, Langerhans cell histiocytosis and lung trauma, including barotrauma.

The natural history of pneumatocoeles is one of spontaneous resolution. Even large pneumatocoeles can resolve in a few days, especially if it is of infective aetiology. Occasionally small thin-walled cysts can be observed for several months following the initial insult; most resolve without sequelae.

A 15-year-old girl develops a diarrhoeal illness with pyrexia. As the diarrhoea is resolving she is noted to be jaundiced. She has pale stools and dark urine. She has a 5 cm liver palpable and a spleen tip. Her liver function tests are as follows:

Bilirubin 198 µmol/l
ALT 1085 U/l
AST 995 U/l
GGT 60 U/l
ALP 785 U/l
Albumin 40 g/l

What further tests would you perform to help make the diagnosis?

SELECT THE *THREE* MOST APPROPRIATE ANSWERS

   i. Viral serology
  ii. Stool for virology
 iii. Abdominal ultrasound scan
  iv. Liver biopsy
   v. Blood gas
  vi. HIDA scan
 vii. Toxicology screen
viii. Ammonia

ANSWERS TO CASE 7.14

  i. Viral serology
 ii. Stool for virology
vii. Toxicology screen

The most likely diagnosis is a viral hepatitis, especially hepatitis A. The other hepatitis viruses, especially B, are also possibilities if she has risk factors. There are many other viruses which also cause acute hepatitis, the most common being EBV, echovirus, coxsackie virus, parvovirus and adenovirus.

In a girl of this age, the possibility of drug toxicity should be considered particularly paracetamol and recreational drugs (ecstasy, solvents, cocaine, etc.).

Factors from the history that should be specifically enquired about include: any history of foreign travel, blood transfusions, i.v. drug abuse, sexual contact, contacts with viral illnesses, overdoses or recreational drugs.

Viral serology and stool for viruses should be sent to help make the diagnosis, as well as a toxicology screen should there be any concerns from the history.

Examination for encephalopathy and measurement of prothrombin time would help ascertain whether she were developing acute liver failure and would need immediate referral to a liver centre. If either of these were abnormal or if there was ongoing concern, the following should be checked: acid–base status, glucose, ammonia, and lactate.

Hepatitis A accounts for 20-25% of acute hepatitis. The picture is typically of hepatitis with some obstructive features. The major complication is acute liver failure which occurs in approximately 0.1% of infected children. Warning signs of progressive disease are grossly elevated transaminases; increased prothrombin time; rapidly increasing bilirubin; decreasing liver size and increasing lethargy/confusion. Once liver failure develops then acid–base derangements, renal compromise, hypoglycaemia and increasing plasma ammonia occur.

Acute abdominal pain may develop, most likely due to acute pancreatitis in both the acute and convalescent phase of hepatitis A, but this could also be due to acute hepatic enlargement or a surgical cause. Investigations would include an ultrasound of liver, biliary tree and pancreas, serum amylase, and possibly a surgical assessment.

A 10-year-old Caucasian girl was found to have proteinuria. She had a 4-year history of rheumatoid factor positive polyarticular juvenile idiopathic arthritis (JIA) that had been treated with weekly i.m. methotrexate over the preceding 3 years. The dose of methotrexate had recently been reduced from 20 mg to 10 mg because of raised hepatic transaminases. Her arthritis is not currently well controlled. There was no history of pre-existing renal disease and no family history of renal problems. Her grandmother had sarcoidosis. On examination, she was normotensive. There was no peripheral oedema. She had evidence of active arthritis in both knees. Remaining examination was unremarkable. Urinalysis showed moderate proteinuria with a protein : creatinine ratio of 200 (normal range <12.5). Serum albumin was in the normal range. There was no biochemical evidence of renal impairment.

Which of the following are not possible causes of the proteinuria?

SELECT *TWO* ANSWERS ONLY

i. Nephrotic syndrome
ii. Methotrexate nephropathy
iii. Sarcoidosis
iv. Renal amyloidosis
v. Interstitial nephritis

ANSWERS TO CASE 7.15

i. Nephrotic syndrome
v. Interstitial nephritis

Polyarticular JIA affects more than four joints in the first 6 months. Rheumatoid factor positive disease typically has a worse prognosis and often requires early treatment with methotrexate. Amyloid proteins can accumulate in any chronic inflammatory condition and may affect up to 10% of children with JIA. Renal amyloidosis may cause isolated proteinuria. There is a family history of sarcoidosis and, although isolated renal involvement is rare, renal sarcoidosis should be considered. Methotrexate has many adverse effects including nephropathy. Proteinuria secondary to methotrexate toxicity must therefore be included in the differential diagnosis. Routine monitoring of patients on methotrexate includes periodic full blood count, hepatic and renal biochemistry, urinalysis and chest radiograph. The clinical picture is not one of nephrotic syndrome. Interstitial nephritis is unlikely in the absence of haematuria.

Proteinuria is a cardinal sign of glomerular disease and, at this level, warrants investigation into the underlying cause. Basic investigation includes renal biochemistry, quantitative urinalysis and a renal tract ultrasound. Results of these along with the clinical history guides further investigation. In this case, the most obvious next investigation is an estimation of serum amyloid protein. Amyloidosis is well recognised in JIA and an important diagnosis to make early. A renal biopsy would differentiate between amyloidosis and methotrexate-induced nephropathy, or suggest an alternative diagnosis. In this case, the serum amyloid A protein was raised at 102 mg/l (normal range <10). Congo red staining of a renal biopsy specimen confirmed glomerular deposition of amyloid protein. Amyloidosis secondary to JIA is classically treated with chlorambucil which may reverse proteinuria and prolong life. In addressing the problem of proteinuria, it is important not to ignore the underlying disease, and with previous hepatic complications of higher dose methotrexate, the options are limited. The TNF-α antagonist Etanercept has recently become available and is being increasingly used as an adjunct to other therapies in the management of JIA.

A female baby was admitted to the paediatric ward at the age of 4 days with a history of vomiting, poor feeding, lethargy and jaundice. She had been born at term to a 29-year-old primigravida, and had had a birth weight of 3120 g. The baby's mother had been well during pregnancy; in the past, she had suffered two generalised seizures but was not taking any medication. The parents were unrelated. There was no family history of jaundice or liver disorder, nor was there any history of sudden neonatal death. The birth had been uncomplicated, and the baby was being breast fed. On examination, she was dehydrated, having lost 13% of her birth weight, and obviously jaundiced. Systemic examination was otherwise unremarkable.

The following tests were carried out:

Total bilirubin 387 µmol/l (conjugated 6)

FBC normal

Blood sugar normal

Direct Coombs' test (DCT) negative

Mother's blood group O positive

Baby's blood group O positive

Urine microscopy normal

Following an initial reduction in the bilirubin level after phototherapy and i.v. fluids, the level rose again and 4 days later was 362 µmol/l (conjugated 79). The baby was well hydrated but had now developed a 3.0 cm hepatomegaly. The stools were pigmented, and eye examination revealed normal bilateral red reflexes. Further phototherapy was given and, as there was a suspicion of a possible metabolic disorder, breast feeds were stopped and a particular formula feed was introduced. This resulted in a dramatic improvement in the infant's condition and a resolution of the jaundice.

What is the most likely diagnosis?

SELECT *ONE* ANSWER ONLY

  i. α-1 antitrypsin deficiency
  ii. Galactosaemia
 iii. Biliary atresia
 iv. Wilson's disease
  v. Niemann–Pick disease

ii. Galactosaemia

The diagnostic clue was that whenever breast feeds were stopped, the baby's condition improved clinically. Classical-form galactosaemia is caused by an inherited deficiency of the enzyme galactose-1-phosphate uridyl transferase (GAL-1-PUT). Further investigations include: LFTs, clotting studies, blood cultures, urine reducing substances, thyroid function tests, glucose-6-phosphate dehydrogenase status, galactase-1-phosphate uridyl transferase activity (Beutler test), urine/blood amino acids and urine organic acids. There is a high risk of E. *coli* septicaemia.

Galactosaemia is an inherited autosomal recessive disorder (1 in 45 000 live-births), most patients being homozygous or heterozygous for Q188R mutation. Deficiency of galactose-1-phosphate uridyl transferase causes accumulation of galactose-1-phosphate in the liver, brain, lenses, kidneys and adrenal glands. If fed lactose (a disaccharide of glucose and galactose), infants present with vomiting, diarrhoea, failure to thrive, developmental delay or retardation, cataracts, jaundice or cirrhosis. Examination may also reveal hepatomegaly, a full fontanelle, bleeding or excessive bruising and evidence of encephalopathy. Biochemical findings are abnormal LFTs, unconjugated or combined hyperbilirubinaemia, abnormal clotting, raised plasma amino acid levels (phenylalanine, tyrosine and methionine), and renal tubular dysfunction leading to aminoaciduria and metabolic acidosis. Preliminary diagnosis is made when reducing substances other than glucose are found in the urine. Diagnosis is confirmed by a low level of GAL-1-PUT in erthyrocytes. Tests include the Beutler test; a widely used fluorescent spot test for galactose-1-phosphate uridyl transferase activity (can use a Guthrie card blood spot). False negatives may occur after blood transfusion. Other tests include an assay of red blood cell galactose-1-phosphate level (not affected by blood transfusion) and DNA analysis (60% of the UK is homozygous for Q188R mutation). Checking the urine for reducing substances is neither sensitive nor specific; small quantities of galactose are often found in the urine of patients with liver disease. Also, galactose may disappear rapidly from the urine in patients with galactosaemia. Initial management is immediate dietary withdrawal of galactose; galactose-free milk substitutes are available on prescription (e.g. infasoy, progestamil). Supportive care may be required. Antibiotics, i.v. fluids and vitamin K are often necessary. Galactose restriction is necessary throughout life to stop any recurrence of severe toxicity. Early treatment does not, however, prevent long-term complications (cognitive dysfunction, and gonadal dysfunction in female patients). Recent evidence suggests there is an endogenous production of galactose that may be responsible for the long-term effects.

Questions and Answers for the New Format Exam

A 12-year-old boy is referred to the growth clinic. His height has fallen from the 90th centile to the 3rd centile between the age of 6 and 12 years. He has no signs of puberty yet. Over the past few months he has had deteriorating school performance and behavioural change. He also complains of paraesthesiae and spasms in his face and arms. While investigations are progressing, he also starts to complain of deteriorating vision, and on ophthalmological examination is found to have bilateral cataracts.

Investigations showed:
Adjusted Ca 0.68 mmol/l
Mg 0.57 mmol/l
PO_4 3.22 mmol/l
Bone age 7 years
EEG generalised slow wave activity of high amplitude
CT head normal

a. What is the next best investigation?
SELECT *ONE* ANSWER ONLY
 i. Parathyroid hormone level
 ii. Vitamin D levels
 iii. Alkaline phosphatase
 iv. DEXA bone scan
 v. X-ray wrist

b. What other conditions may be associated with this boy's diagnosis?
SELECT THE *THREE* BEST ANSWERS
 i. Ectodermal dysplasia
 ii. Congenital heart disease
 iii. Eczema
 iv. Alopecia
 v. Addison's disease
 vi. Hypothyroidism
 vii. Renal osteodystrophy
 viii. Cleft palate

ANSWERS TO CASE 7.17

a.   i. Parathyroid hormone levels
b.   i. Ectodermal dysplasia
    iv. Alopecia
    v. Addison's disease

This boy has hypoparathyroidism. The cataracts have developed as a result of severe hypocalcaemia. Hypocalcaemia is also the cause of his abnormal EEG, and his tetanic spasms. ECG changes are also likely to occur with severe hypocalcaemia, typically a prolonged QT interval.

Parathyroid hormone levels need to be checked to confirm the probable diagnosis of hypoparathyroidism. In this child they were very low at 0.1 pmol/l. Typical laboratory findings in hypoparathyroidism are low calcium, raised phosphate, normal or low alkaline phosphatase, low parathyroid hormone and low vitamin D.

The hypocalcaemia needs to be slowly corrected. This will require a calcium and vitamin D therapy, with careful monitoring for calcium toxicity (nephrocalcinosis, and nephrolithiasis). A suggested scheme is:

- Acute calcium supplementation with i.v. calcium gluconate 0.3 ml/kg of 10% injection, diluted five-fold and given slowly. Monitor for bradycardia and extravasation
- Calcium supplement 1 mmol/kg/day orally
- Alfacalcidol (1-alpha-hydroxycholecalciferol) 0.05 µg/kg/day starting dose
- Calcitriol (1,25-dihydroxycholecalciferol) initially 250 ng/day (short-acting therefore will not slowly accumulate and cause delayed vitamin D toxicity)
- Hypomagnesaemia needs correction.

Hypoparathyroidism in childhood is usually autoimmune. It is associated with muco-cutaneous candidiasis and Addison's disease. Other associated conditions are alopecia, diabetes mellitus and ectodermal dysplasia. When these associations are present, it constitutes autoimmune polyendocrinopathy 1 or the APECED syndrome. Antibodies targeting the calcium sensing receptor can be identified. Patients have concurrent steatorrhoea and low magnesium levels.

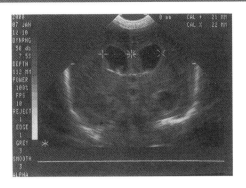

Fig 7.18

A 2-week-old baby presented clinically septic. He was born at term, and had been well until 24 h before admission. Analysis of his CSF showed 285 × 10⁶/l WBC (90% polymorphs), 1000 × 10⁶/l red blood cells, protein 4.9 g/dl and glucose 1.9 mmol/l. Subsequent CSF and blood cultures were positive for *E. coli*, sensitive to cefotaxime, with which he was treated from admission. After 1 week of treatment he was still spiking high temperatures, and remained lethargic with poor feeding. A cerebral ultrasound was performed and is shown.

a. What complication has occurred?
  SELECT *ONE* ANSWER ONLY
  i. Cerebellar coning
  ii. Acute hydrocephalus
  iii. Intraventricular haemorrhage
  iv. Ependymal cyst
  v. Periventricular leukomalacia

b. What further investigations are required?
  SELECT *TWO* ANSWERS ONLY
  i. CT scan
  ii. Intraventricular tap
  iii. MRI
  iv. Repeat lumbar puncture
  v. ECG

ANSWERS TO CASE 7.18

a. ii. Acute hydrocephalus
b. i. CT scan
   iv. Repeat lumbar puncture

The diagnosis here is neonatal meningitis secondary to *E. coli* infection. The complication is acute hydrocephalus and probably ventriculitis. Further investigations would include a CT scan, repeat lumbar puncture to send CSF for further culture and sensitivity, and neurosurgical referral for decompression of the hydrocephalus.

Options include:
- repeated percutaneous ventricular taps
- insertion of a reservoir, e.g. an Ommaya reservoir, through which repeated ventricular taps can be performed and, if desired, intraventricular antibiotics given
- percutaneous endoscopic third and fourth ventriculostomies, to encourage CSF flow and removal
- ventriculo–peritoneal (VP) shunt

Hydrocephalus is an acute complication of meningitis, uncommon beyond the neonatal period. The incidence has greatly reduced over the years with the use of improved antibiotics. Gram-negative organisms are most commonly associated with hydrocephalus formation. The experience of some neurosurgeons is that ventriculostomy has decreased the need for a VP shunt by one-third. In this case, his repeat CSF samples showed $1600 \times 10^6/l$ WBC (90% polymorphs), $1000 \times 10^6/l$ red blood cells, with again a positive culture for *E. coli* sensitive to cefotaxime indicating a ventriculitis. He underwent reservoir insertion, then ventriculostomies, but eventually had a VP shunt insertion.

6, 8

CASE 7.19

1. Von–Hippel–Lindau syndrome
2. Lennox–Gastaut syndrome
3. Abetalipoproteinaemia
4. Leigh syndrome
5. Marchiafava–Bignami syndrome
6. Joubert's syndrome
7. Niemann–Pick disease
8. West syndrome
9. Neuronal migration disorder
10. Multiple sclerosis

For each of the following case scenarios select the most likely diagnosis from the list above;

a. A 4-week-old baby presented with intermittent tachypnoea and apnoea since day 1 of life. Episodes were multiple each day and mostly self-resolving, though mild stimulation would be required occasionally. Associated with the apnoea she would become cyanosed. She was otherwise well and was feeding orally. She had no constant oxygen requirement.

The baby was born at full term by normal vaginal delivery. There was no resuscitation at birth. Family history was negative for congenital abnormalities and neurological disorders. Examination revealed a non-dysmorphic child with axial hypotonia and erratic nystagmus and dysconjugate eye movements. The rest of the neurological examination was normal. MRI showed an absent cerebellar vermis, and the characteristic "molar tooth" sign on axial images.

b. A 5-year-old girl with "dystonic cerebral palsy" presented with a 4-week history of respiratory difficulty. Initially this had been associated with a respiratory tract infection, but over the 4-week period a disordered respiratory pattern had emerged. She had a normal birth to unrelated parents but was developmentally delayed at the age of 6 months. At this time her parents had also noted breath-holding episodes with loss of consciousness. Examination revealed dystonic posture with stiffness and hyperreflexia of her limbs, truncal hypotonia, fine nystagmus and tremor on movement. She had pale optic discs, but vision seemed unimpaired. A brain MRI at this time demonstrated mild atrophy and her condition appeared to be static.

c. A 3-day-old female infant on the post-natal ward had been noted to be feeding poorly since birth and the midwife is concerned that she was floppy. She had a couple of twitchy episodes which resolved spontaneously. Her blood glucose had been normal. Antenatal scans showed polyhydramnios but were otherwise normal. She is the first child of unrelated Caucasian parents. On examination, she has mild dysmorphic features including a high forehead with central furrowing, bitemporal narrowing and bilateral 5th finger clinodactyly. Her weight is on the 25th centile and her head circumference on the 9th centile. She is centrally hypotonic and has a poor suck. A cranial USS shows few visible gyri, and an EEG is performed showing hypsarrthymia.

a. 6. Joubert's syndrome

Joubert's syndrome is a clinical presentation of episodic apnoea/tachypnoea with nystagmus, ataxia, developmental delay and cerebellar vermian dysgenesis. MRI is characteristic and differentiates it from Dandy–Walker malformation. Abnormal breathing pattern has been reported in the majority of cases and occurs in both REM and non-REM sleep as well as whilst awake. The exact aetiology is unknown. A proportion of patients will have retinal dystrophy. Some patients are severely affected and die in infancy. The majority of those who survive have delayed development and learning difficulties.

b. 4. Leigh syndrome

Leigh syndrome is a progressive neurodegenerative condition of infancy and childhood. It is thought to result from a severe failure of oxidative metabolism within mitochondria of the developing brain. Inheritance can be X-linked recessive or autosomal recessive depending on the defect responsible. The characteristic symmetric necrotic lesions distributed along the brainstem, diencephalons and basal ganglia are readily visible on MRI or CT, but may not be present on scans in early life. The clinical presentation and course may vary considerably but symptoms often include signs of brainstem or basal ganglia dysfunction. Developmental delay and regression are prominent clinical features of this disorder. The clinical course can follow a stepwise deterioration with some recovery of developmental skills between episodes of regression or a slowly progressive decline. Investigations include cerebral imaging, muscle biopsy and CSF lactate (may be raised, but normal levels do not exclude the diagnosis).

c. 9. Neuronal migration disorder

Neuronal migration disorders are malformations of cortical development, and are highly associated with epilepsy, developmental delay and mental retardation. Associated features may include autism, learning difficulties, hypotonia and spasticity. In some cases, there is global neurodevastation and failure to thrive. This baby had Miller–Dieker syndrome, a neuronal migration disorder, as suggested by her clinical features and lissencephaly (smooth brain) which can be confirmed on MRI. These patients need to be managed by a multi-disciplinary team. They often fail to thrive, and require gastrostomy feeding. A paediatric neurologist should be involved if seizures are intractable. Death usually occurs before 2 years of age. A deletion of 17p13.3 has been documented in the majority of cases. Hypsarrythmia refers to a chaotic EEG with high-amplitude asymmetrical non-synchronous spike, polyspike and slow waves, with an irregular background activity. Treatment of hypsarrythmia is difficult and resistant to most antiepileptic drugs. Recently, vigabatrin has been used successfully, but it can cause visual field defects which are irreversible.

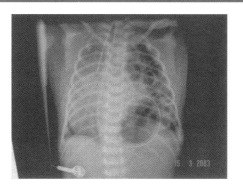

Fig 7.20

You have been called to see a newborn baby aged 40 min on the neonatal unit. Born at 34 weeks' gestation with an insignificant antenatal history, he was put on CPAP because of mild respiratory distress. The nurses report that the oxygen saturation had dropped from 95% in air to 78% in 45% oxygen. On examination, the respiratory rate is 60/min with some intercostal recession and reduced air entry on the left. The urgent CXR is shown.

What is the diagnosis?

SELECT *ONE* ANSWER ONLY

   i. Left-sided pneumothorax
  ii. Left-sided pneumatocoles
 iii. Congenital pulmonary emphysema
  iv. Congenital cystic malformation of the lung
   v. Left-sided congenital diaphragmatic hernia
  vi. Loculated empyema

ANSWER TO CASE 7.20

v. Left-sided congenital diaphragmatic hernia

The CXR shows fluid levels in the left hemithorax, an abnormal position of the nasogastric tube, and mediastinal shift to the right all consistent with a diagnosis of left-sided diaphragmatic hernia.

Congenital diaphragmatic hernia (CDH) occurs in one of every 2000-4000 live births and accounts for 8% of all major congenital anomalies. The risk of recurrence of isolated CDH for future siblings is approximately 2%. Infants may have an antenatal history of polyhydramnios and most commonly present with a history of cyanosis and respiratory distress in the first minutes or hours of life, although a later presentation is possible. They frequently exhibit a scaphoid abdomen.

Chapter

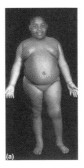 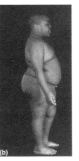

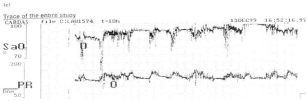

Fig 8.1

This 5-year-old boy presented with a history of marked snoring every night, shortness of breath on exertion and excessive day-time sleepiness. He has been diagnosed with Prader–Willi syndrome.

a. What investigation was performed (Fig. 8.1.c)?
SELECT *ONE* ANSWER ONLY
  i. Cardiotocograph
 ii. Sleep study
iii. Exercise ECG
 iv. Spirometry
  v. Pulse oximetry

b. What does the result show?
SELECT *THE BEST* ANSWER ONLY
  i. REM sleep pattern
 ii. Oxygen desaturations
iii. Obstructive airways disease
 iv. Right heart strain
  v. Obstructive sleep apnoea

c. What other investigations would you request for this patient?
SELECT *TWO* ANSWERS ONLY
  i. CT head
 ii. ECG
iii. Bone scan
 iv. Echocardiogram
  v. Glucose tolerance test

ANSWERS TO CASE 8.1

a. v. Pulse oximetry
b. v. Obstructive sleep apnoea
c. ii. ECG
    iv. Echocardiogram

Prader–Willi syndrome is inherited by uniparental maternal disomy on chromosome 15. The characteristic features include: fetal and infantile hypotonia, small hands and feet, post-natally acquired obesity through voracious appetite, cryptorchidism, micropenis and mild mental retardation. Excessive daytime sleepiness occurs in approximately 50-75% of patients with Prader–Willi syndrome. Children with this syndrome have been shown to have increased number of apnoeas, a decreased nadir of oxygen saturation, and decreased respiratory response to hypercapnia during quiet sleep. Obstructive sleep apnoea is one important factor related to subsequent daytime sleepiness, worsened by obesity. An additional central disturbance sleep mechanism (hypothalamic dysfunction) is thought to be present.

Investigations include pulse oximetry, which in this example shows episodes of severe desaturations down to around 65% during REM sleep (with a corresponding rise in heart rate). This pattern is consistent with obstructive sleep apnoea.

An ECG is done to look for right ventricular hypertrophy, and an echocardiogram to exclude right heart failure.

Treatments are symptomatic. Adenotonsillectomy may be beneficial, but does not consistently cure all symptoms. Weight loss should be encouraged. CPAP may be used during sleep, but, in severe cases, an artificial airway may be required, e.g. nasopharyngeal tube or tracheostomy. Diuretics may be needed to relieve right heart failure as an adjunctive therapy.

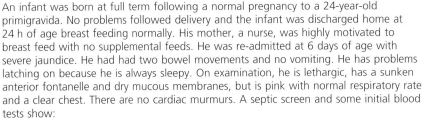

An infant was born at full term following a normal pregnancy to a 24-year-old primigravida. No problems followed delivery and the infant was discharged home at 24 h of age breast feeding normally. His mother, a nurse, was highly motivated to breast feed with no supplemental feeds. He was re-admitted at 6 days of age with severe jaundice. He had had two bowel movements and no vomiting. He has problems latching on because he is always sleepy. On examination, he is lethargic, has a sunken anterior fontanelle and dry mucous membranes, but is pink with normal respiratory rate and a clear chest. There are no cardiac murmurs. A septic screen and some initial blood tests show:

Na 170 mmol/l
K 4.2 mmol/l
Creatinine 105 μmol/l
Cl 130 mmol/l
Ca 2.2 mmol/l
Total bilirubin 425 μmol/l
Hb 22 g/dl
WCC 14 × 10⁹/l
Platelets 359 × 10⁹/l

a. What is the other most useful measurement?
SELECT *ONE* ANSWER ONLY
i. Serum osmolality
ii. Urea
iii. Urine osmolality
iv. Weight of baby
v. Blood gas

b. What is the most likely cause of the biochemical abnormalities?
SELECT *ONE* ANSWER ONLY
i. Renal dysfunction with polyuria
ii. Diabetes insipidus
iii. Intake of over-concentrated feeds
iv. Inadequate breast feeding
v. Cystic fibrosis

c. Which of the following are likely to be involved in treatment?
SELECT *TWO* ANSWERS ONLY
i. i.v. normal saline
ii. i.v. 10% dextrose
iii. Oral rehydration with water
iv. Oral rehydration with electrolyte solution
v. i.v. bolus of normal saline
vi. Oral rehydration with milk
vii. i.v. 10% dextrose with electrolytes

ANSWERS TO CASE 8.2

a. iv. Weight of baby
b. iv. Inadequate breast feeding
c. vi. Oral rehydration with milk
   vii. i.v. 10% dextrose with electrolytes

Weighing the infant reveals that he has lost 25% of his birthweight indicating that the hypernatraemia and hyperbilirubinaemia are due to dehydration.

It is likely that this baby's hypernatraemic dehydration is due to inadequate breast milk intake. Despite its proven advantages, there are complications of breast feeding. Loss of water from insensible losses through the skin and lungs in the absence of concomitant sodium loss without adequate intake may result in this picture.

This infant had hypernatraemic dehydration due to inadequate intake secondary to a poor breast milk supply. The most important treatment is slow rehydration. The fluid deficit is calculated from the weight loss and replaced over 48 h to prevent too rapid a fall in the serum sodium concentration; i.v. treatment is given as 10% dextrose with normal sodium content (3-4 mmol/kg/day). Ideally, breast feeding should be continued but additional support and monitoring will be required. As the infant is rehydrated, the serum bilirubin will also fall back into the normal range, but phototherapy should also be used to help decrease the bilirubin concentration.

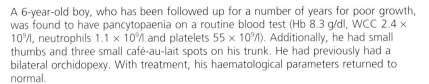
CASE 8.3

A 6-year-old boy, who has been followed up for a number of years for poor growth, was found to have pancytopaenia on a routine blood test (Hb 8.3 g/dl, WCC 2.4 × 10^9/l, neutrophils 1.1 × 10^9/l and platelets 55 × 10^9/l). Additionally, he had small thumbs and three small café-au-lait spots on his trunk. He had previously had a bilateral orchidopexy. With treatment, his haematological parameters returned to normal.

Six months later, he developed a vesicular, painful rash in a dermatomal distribution in the right lumbar area.

a. Suggest the underlying diagnosis, and a way of confirming it:
   SELECT *ONE* ANSWER ONLY
   i. Holt–Oram syndrome
   ii. Pseudohypoparathyroidism
   iii. Hypoparathyroidism
   iv. Fanconi's anaemia
   v. Neurofibromatosis

b. Name one important long-term complication:
   SELECT *ONE* ANSWER ONLY
   i. Splenomegaly
   ii. Aplastic anaemia
   iii. Malignancy
   iv. Neurological manifestations
   v. Pneumococcal infection

ANSWERS TO CASE 8.3

a. iv. Fanconi's anaemia
b. iii. Malignancy

Pancytopaenia with small thumbs, café-au-lait spots and poor growth suggests a diagnosis of Fanconi's anaemia. This is an autosomal recessive disorder of DNA repair, with a high risk of malignancies, and renal dysfunction. Without treatment, the average life span is approximately 15 years. Bone marrow transplantation is curative if successful, but immunosuppression makes overwhelming varicella infection a serious risk.

Confirmation of the diagnosis of Fanconi's anaemia is made by a chromosome fragility test.

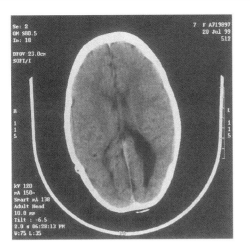

Fig 8.4

A 9-year-old girl is referred from the ophthalmology clinic. Her visual acuity is 6/12 in the right eye and 6/18 in the left eye. Her optic discs are pale. She was born at 31 weeks' gestation the first of twins. She required ventilation for the first week and developed an intra-ventricular haemorrhage with secondary hydrocephalus requiring a shunt at 5 months of age. Her fine motor skills are slightly behind those of her peers and sister but she attends mainstream school. A CT brain scan was arranged (Fig. 8.4).

What abnormality is shown?

SELECT *ONE* ANSWER ONLY
  i. Right sided mass in posterior ventricle
  ii. Cystic periventricular leukomalacia
  iii. Hydrocephalus
  iv. Left intraventricular haemorrhage
  v. Non-cystic periventricular leukomalacia

ANSWER TO CASE 8.4

iv. Non-cystic periventricular leukomalacia

The CT shows periventricular leukomalacia (PVL) or white matter loss in the posterior temporal and parietal lobes, in this case non-cystic.

The child's reduced visual acuity is likely to be a complication of her preterm birth, although there are many theoretical causes. This child may have had retinopathy of prematurity in the past, or her pale optic discs may represent optic atrophy secondary to hydrocephalus. Periventricular leukomalacia may also be the cause of her reduced vision since development of neonatal vision is subcortically mediated and lesions affecting the optic radiations, especially cystic PVL, may subsequently affect visual acuity.

These appearances on the CT scan could also be associated with cerebral palsy (especially spastic diplegia) and other visual problems such as visual field defects, non-paralytic strabismus, oculomotor dyspraxia, optokinetic nystagmus and reduced binocular visual acuity.

CASE 8.5

A 5-year-old girl presented with pubic hair development. She had been born at 36 weeks' gestation weighing 1800 g. She was otherwise healthy. On examination her height was on the 90th centile. She had acneiform lesions on the forehead. There was no breast development; there was sparse pubic hair and some cliteromegaly.

Her serum electrolytes were: Na 137 mmol/l, K 4.0 mmol/l, urea 4.4 mmol/l and creatinine 52 μmol/l.

a. What possible diagnoses should be considered?
SELECT *TWO* ANSWERS ONLY
   i. Precocious puberty
  ii. Congenital adrenal hyperplasia
 iii. Testicular feminisation syndrome
  iv. Cushing's syndrome
   v. Craniopharyngioma

b. What additional investigations are indicated?
SELECT *TWO* ANSWERS ONLY
   i. 17-OHP
  ii. Urinary steroid profile
 iii. LH/FSH
  iv. CT head
   v. Serum testosterone

ANSWERS TO CASE 8.5

a. ii. Congenital adrenal hyperplasia
    iv. Cushing's syndrome
b. i. 17-OHP
    ii. Urinary steroid profile

These signs are due to excess androgen production. Causes include congenital adrenal hyperplasia, adrenal tumour, ectopic androgen-secreting tumours (e.g. teratoma) and Cushing's syndrome. This girl is showing pseudo-precocious puberty, i.e. there is a lack of consonance in pubertal development. The clitoral enlargement makes simple premature adrenarche unlikely.

Investigations should include 17-hydroxyprogesterone, cortisol (0900 and 2400), urinary steroid profile, ultrasound of adrenals and ovaries, X-ray of left wrist for bone age, and renin and aldosterone.

In this case, the urinary steroid profile was diagnostic, showing the characteristic pattern of 21-hydroxylase deficiency, with increased metabolites of 17-hydroxyprogesterone and an increase of androgen metabolites relative to cortisol metabolites. One quarter of children with 21-hydroxylase deficiency are non salt-wasting. The bone age in this girl was characteristically advanced at 8.1 years.

Treatment is with hydrocortisone, initially 20 mg/m^2/day, in three divided doses. The dose is adjusted according to subsequent profiles of 17-hydroxyprogesterone and assessment of growth and bone age. The child may need to be seen by a paediatric urologist and may require cliteroplasty.

Inheritance of congenital adrenal hyperplasia is autosomal recessive, therefore both parents are carriers. The girl had an elder sister whose urine steroid profile was normal. No further children were planned (antenatal diagnosis and treatment of affected female pregnancies with dexamethasone can be offered).

CASE 8.6

A previously fit and well 14-year-old girl presented with a 7-week history of malaise and lethargy, associated with constipation and abdominal pain. On assessment, she was unwell and pale. Her abdomen was distended and tender. She had two small aphthous ulcers in her mouth and three ulcerated skin lesions over both elbows. Investigations showed a microcytic anaemia and an elevated ESR and CRP. Her abdominal radiograph showed faecal loading.

a. **What is the most likely diagnosis?**
   SELECT THE *BEST* ANSWER
   i. Irritable bowel syndrome
   ii. Lymphoma
   iii. Crohn's disease
   iv. Wegener's granulomatosis
   v. Ovarian carcinoma
   vi. Hypothyroidism

b. **What further investigations are required?**
   SELECT THE *TWO* BEST ANSWERS
   i. Barium meal and follow-through
   ii. LFTs
   iii. CT abdomen
   iv. White cell scan
   v. Thyroid function tests
   vi. Autoimmune screen
   vii. Bone marrow aspirate

ANSWERS TO CASE 8.6

a. iii. Crohn's disease
b. i. Barium meal and follow-through
    iv. White cell scan

The onset of Crohn's disease is often insidious. Cramping abdominal pain, weight loss and diarrhoea are common manifestations. The patient may also have fever or constipation. There are many extra-intestinal manifestations such as polyarticular arthritis, pericholangitis, hepatitis, sacroileitis, skin lesions and iritis which may precede gastrointestinal disease. Perianal disease may produce fissures, fistulas or abscesses. The pathology of Crohn's disease involves non-caseating granuloma formation in a discontinuous pattern (skipped lesions) and transmural inflammation in the ileum and colon. The differential diagnosis includes chronic bacterial or parasitic infection such as giardiasis and yersinia enterocolitica.

Investigations that should be performed include a barium meal and follow-through, a colonoscopy and a white cell scan.

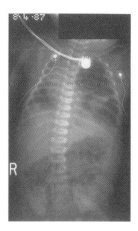

Fig 8.7

This baby was born at 35 weeks' gestation by elective Caesarean section. Severe respiratory failure was evident from birth and ventilation was required. The CXR done at 1 h of age is shown.

What is the most likely diagnosis?

SELECT *ONE* ANSWER ONLY
   i. Cystic fibrosis
  ii. Left pneumothorax
 iii. Staphylococcal sepsis
 iv. Cystic adenomatoid malformation of the lung
  v. Left diaphragmatic hernia

ANSWER TO CASE 8.7

iv. Cystic adenomatoid malformation of the lung

This baby has a cystic adenomatoid malformation of the left lung. The main differential diagnosis is a left diaphragmatic hernia. The key to making the correct diagnosis is noting that the stomach and bowel are in the normal position. If in doubt, for instance when the stomach has no gas in it, a small amount of contrast material can be inserted into the stomach to define its position.

If the baby is asymptomatic, the lesion is usually removed electively when the child is older.

CASE 8.8

A baby girl was born at 35 weeks' gestation to consanguineous parents following polyhydramnios and symmetrical intrauterine growth retardation in pregnancy.

Obstetric history: One previous child was born at term with no problems; the mother had had three miscarriages for no known reason.

After birth there was an uneventful initial course, but at 8 days of age she had lost 15% of her birth weight. She had been tolerating feeds well and there had been no diarrhoea or vomiting. Examination, apart from symmetrical growth retardation, was normal including blood pressure. Blood urea, creatinine and electrolytes were as follows:

Na 113 mmol/l
K 1.8 mmol/l
Cl 60 mmol/l
Bicarbonate 38 mmol/l
Urea 10.1 mmol/l
Creatinine 55 μmol/l
Urinary Cl 32 mmol/l

What is the diagnosis?

SELECT *ONE* ANSWER ONLY

i. Renal tubular acidosis type II
ii. Neonatal Bartter syndrome
iii. Acute tubular necrosis
iv. Congenital adrenal hyperplasia
v. Acute renal failure
vi. Renal tubular acidosis type I

ANSWER TO CASE 8.8

ii. Neonatal Bartter syndrome

The biochemical abnormality is a hypokalaemic hypochloraemic metabolic alkalosis with hyponatraemia. Conditions associated with hypokalaemic hypochloraemic metabolic alkalosis and normal blood pressure can be differentiated on the basis of urinary chloride excretion. In those with extra-renal losses of chloride (gastrointestinal or sweat), the normal kidneys respond by reducing urinary chloride excretion (<10 mmol/l). In this situation, a high urinary chloride excretion (>20 mmol/l) suggested a renal loss of chloride and therefore either Bartter-like syndrome or diuretic use/abuse. Detection of diuretics in the urine, if required, helps establish the difference. U&E should be sent to confirm the renal loss of electrolytes. In this case, there was also increased urinary sodium, potassium and calcium. A capillary gas should be checked to confirm metabolic alkalosis (demonstrated by the high bicarbonate). Renin and aldosterone would be elevated. The hypokalaemia promotes aldosterone secretion and increased prostaglandin production promotes secretion of renin and further increased aldosterone production.

Bartter syndrome represents a closely related set of renal tubular disorders characterised by hypokalaemia, hypochloraemia, metabolic alkalosis and hyperreninaemia with normal BP. The underlying renal abnormality results in excessive urinary losses of sodium, potassium and chloride. Bartter syndrome can be divided into neonatal and classic types.

Neonatal (or pre-natal) Bartter or Hyperprostaglandin E syndrome (HPGES) is characterised by polyhydramnios due to intrauterine polyuria, premature delivery and growth retardation. They often have specific facies: a triangular-shaped face, prominent forehead, large eyes, protruding ears and a drooping mouth. BP is normal. Life-threatening episodes of fever and dehydration during the early weeks of life may occur, due to massive neonatal polyuria (urine output up to 50 ml/kg/h). The essential features include hypokalaemic hypochloraemic metabolic alkalosis, normal blood pressure, increased urinary potassium and chloride loss and elevated plasma renin and aldosterone. Defective maximal concentration and dilution of urine, hypercalciuria, hypomagnesaemia, osteopaenia, increased urinary prostaglandins are also present.

Classic Bartter syndrome. Patients have a history of maternal polyhydramnios and premature delivery. Symptoms in classic Bartter syndrome include polyuria, polydipsia, vomiting, constipation, salt craving, failure to thrive, and in late childhood, fatigue, muscle cramps, recurrent carpopedal spasms. There may be developmental delay and minimal brain dysfunction. Facial appearance may be similar to that of neonatal Bartter, but this is infrequent. Genetic mutations (chromosome15q) lead to defective transepithelial chloride transport across the thick ascending limb (TAL) of the loop of Henlé. The resultant decrease in sodium chloride reabsorption in the TAL will reduce medullary hypertonicity, perhaps explaining the concentrating defect. With the markedly increased salt delivery to the distal nephron, sodium is exchanged for potassium. Increased sodium reabsorption via the epithelial channel, coupled with increased potassium and hydrogen ion secretion in the collecting tubule would cause hypokalaemic metabolic alkalosis. The markedly increased salt delivery to the distal nephron causes salt wasting, volume contraction and stimulation of the renin-angiotensin-aldosterone axis. Impaired electrogenic chloride transport in the TAL also inhibits the voltage drive, paracellular reabsorption of calcium and magnesium and thus causes hypercalciuria and magnesuria. Hypokalaemia, chronic volume contraction and elevated levels of angiotensin, kallikrein, kinins and vasopressin all stimulate prostaglandin E2 production. This and chronic volume contraction probably cause the resistance to the pressor effects of angiotensin or catecholamines and this may explain the normal blood pressure in the presence of elevated renin levels.

CASE 8.9

A 4-year-old-boy was referred to outpatients after two generalised afebrile tonic clonic seizures lasting up to 10 min. A 6-month history of frequent falls was elicited which were causing concerns at nursery and were used as the explanation for his bruises. These falls would happen several times a day, his eyes would roll back and he would fall to the ground for up to 4 min with no aura or warning. In between falls, he was well. His past medical history included a minor head injury.

He was delayed in reaching his milestones but there was no history of regression. Examination revealed microcephaly and multiple bruises. An EEG showed a slow polyrhythmical background with high-voltage irregular delta waves in the anterior region, and frequent bursts of generalised irregular spike and wave activity. Upon review in outpatients, he had developed myoclonic seizures.

a. What is the diagnosis?
   SELECT THE MOST APPROPRIATE ANSWER
   i. Wiskott–Aldrich syndrome
   ii. Lennox–Gastaut syndrome
   iii. Rett's syndrome
   iv. West syndrome
   v. Angelman syndrome
   vi. Acute demyelinating encephalomyelitis

b. Which anticonvulsant would you start?
   SELECT ONE ANSWER ONLY
   i. Vigabatrin
   ii. Sodium valproate
   iii. Carbamazepine
   iv. Phenobarbitone
   v. Lamotrigine

ANSWERS TO CASE 8.9

a. ii. Lennox–Gastaut syndrome
b. ii. Sodium valproate

Lennox–Gastaut syndrome is a severe form of childhood epilepsy characterised by multiple seizure types (tonic, atonic/drop attacks, myoclonic, atypical absences), developmental delay, behavioural disturbances and a characteristic EEG. The incidence is one in 10 000. It usually develops between the ages of 3 and 5 years. Sixty per cent of children with the syndrome have neurological symptoms prior to the onset of seizures, and the majority have intellectual impairment at diagnosis. Behavioural disturbances such as poor social skills and attention-seeking behaviour are common. In 30% of cases, there is a history of infantile spasms. The prognosis is usually poor. Nearly 80% continue with seizures in adult life, and only 17% can lead independent lives. Sodium valproate is the initial anti-epileptic medication of choice, as carbamazepine may increase the frequency of myoclonic seizures. Two-thirds of patients will be resistant to conventional therapy.

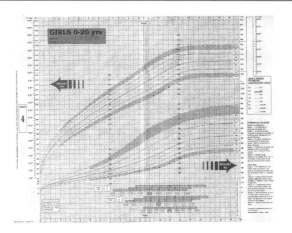

Fig 8.10

A 13-year-old girl was referred to the endocrine clinic, as her parents were concerned about her short stature. She was in good health and was developmentally normal. Her parents described her appetite as poor but her diet was said to be healthy. On examination, she had a few pigmented naevi and low set ears but had no other specific dysmorphic features. She was noted to have an ejection systolic murmur grade 2/6, maximal at the left sternal edge. Her blood pressure was 100/60, and her peripheral pulses were normal. Her growth chart is shown. Her mid-parental height was 169 cm. She was pre-pubertal.

What initial investigations should be performed?

SELECT THE *THREE* MOST APPROPRIATE ANSWERS

  i. CXR
 ii. Thyroid function tests
iii. Bone age
 iv. FBC
  v. Coeliac screen
 vi. Karyotype
vii. CT brain
viii. LH/FSH

ii. Thyroid function tests
iii. Bone age
vi. Karyotype

Investigations should include a karyotype, thyroid function tests, U&E, blood glucose, LFTs, FBC, ESR, calcium, phosphate, ALP, bone age, echocardiography, and possibly a coeliac screen.

The diagnosis in this girl was Turner's syndrome. She has a karyotype of 45 XO, with no evidence of mosaicism. The diagnosis should be considered in any girl with unexplained short stature whether or not there are any suggestive phenotypic features. Turner's syndrome occurs with a frequency of approximately 1 in 2500 live births. Two-thirds of cases have the 45 XO genotype, the remaining one-third have a mosaic chromosome pattern or loss of only a part of the X chromosome. Twenty-four per cent have cryptic Y chromosome material. In girls with Turner's syndrome it is important to obtain a cardiology opinion, whether or not they have signs suggestive of an underlying cardiac problem. There is a recognised mortality from cardiovascular malformations (coarctation, aortic dilatation, dissection or rupture) in young adulthood.

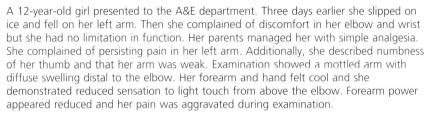

CASE 8.11

A 12-year-old girl presented to the A&E department. Three days earlier she slipped on ice and fell on her left arm. Then she complained of discomfort in her elbow and wrist but she had no limitation in function. Her parents managed her with simple analgesia. She complained of persisting pain in her left arm. Additionally, she described numbness of her thumb and that her arm was weak. Examination showed a mottled arm with diffuse swelling distal to the elbow. Her forearm and hand felt cool and she demonstrated reduced sensation to light touch from above the elbow. Forearm power appeared reduced and her pain was aggravated during examination.

What is the likeliest diagnosis?

SELECT *ONE* ANSWER ONLY

  i. Ulnar nerve dysfunction
 ii. Compartment syndrome
iii. Reflex sympathetic dystrophy
 iv. Radial nerve dysfunction
  v. Supracondylar fracture with associated peripheral neuropathy
 vi. Inflammatory mononeuritis

ANSWER TO CASE 8.11

iii. Reflex sympathetic dystrophy

Reflex sympathetic dystrophy (RSD), also known as complex regional pain syndrome (CRPS), is a clinical diagnosis, but X-rays, Doppler studies and bone scintigraphy are perhaps the most appropriate investigations to rule out other pathologies. Treatment involves firm reassurance supported by intensive physiotherapy, perhaps augmented by simple analgesia. Normal use of the affected limb should be strongly encouraged. Immobilising the limb in response to discomfort is unhelpful and may exacerbate the condition. Underlying psychological factors may be involved, so referral for child and family psychiatry evaluation should be considered. RSD/CRPS appears less common in children than in adults, but can cause significant morbidity. The diagnosis can be made in the context of a history of trauma to the affected area, with pain and mobility disturbance disproportionate to the initial injury. Delayed recognition means that many children undergo extensive investigations to rule out a wide range of possible underlying conditions. Any skin stimulation, such as water in a shower, may be perceived as painful (allodynia). Other features include:

- Sympathetic disturbance – changes in skin temperature, increased sweating, colour changes (mottling/pallor/blue) due to vasomotor changes
- Swelling – diffuse oedema often localized to the painful area
- Movement disturbance – from pain, stiffness and true difficulty in initiating muscle movement
- Changes in tissue growth (dystrophy)

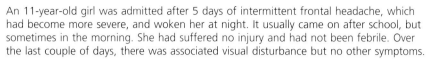
An 11-year-old girl was admitted after 5 days of intermittent frontal headache, which had become more severe, and woken her at night. It usually came on after school, but sometimes in the morning. She had suffered no injury and had not been febrile. Over the last couple of days, there was associated visual disturbance but no other symptoms.

Her past history included severe asthma, requiring long-term inhaled steroids, and short stature, with bone age delay. Anterior pituitary function testing, including an insulin tolerance test, had shown growth hormone insufficiency, a pre-pubertal LHRH response, a good cortisol response, and normal baseline thyroid function. Cranial MRI, to exclude a tumour, was normal. Growth hormone had therefore been started. Examination demonstrated no meningism, and no focal neurological signs. Visual fields, acuity and colour vision were all normal. However, she had papilloedema.

Lumbar puncture revealed pressure of 24 cm of water, no white cells, two red cells, protein of 15 mg/dl and glucose of 4 mmol/l.

What is the diagnosis?

SELECT *ONE* ANSWER ONLY

  i. Craniopharyngioma
  ii. Viral encephalitis
 iii. Subacute sclerosing panencephalitis
 iv. Acute demyelinating encephalitis
  v. Benign intracranial hypertension (BIH)

ANSWER TO CASE 8.12

iii. Benign intracranial hypertension (BIH)

BIH (also known as pseudotumour cerebri) is characterised by signs and symptoms of increased intracranial pressure with no evidence of underlying systemic causes. Symptoms include headache, nausea and vomiting, blurred vision and diplopia. Loss of vision is a serious complication. The diagnosis is suggested by the presence of papilloedema, a sixth nerve palsy, and a raised opening CSF pressure (with no ventricular dilatation).

The aetiology of the increased CSF pressure is not known. Theories include obstruction to the flow of CSF at the arachnoid granulations, an increased rate of CSF formation, changes in the brain parenchyma and blood vessels, obstruction to venous outflow at the superior sagittal sinus and a reduced ability of the subarachnoid space to expand. Initial management involves removing CSF by lumbar puncture to bring pressure below 20 cm.

Many causes have been implicated in BIH: endocrine (e.g. Addison's, hypothyroidism, hyperthyroidism, hypoparathyroidism); drugs (e.g. vitamin A, retinoids, tetracyclines, thyroxine, growth hormone, corticosteroids [and their withdrawal], nitrofurantoin and lithium); viral infections; Lyme disease; iron deficiency anaemia; trauma; and idiopathic (the most common).

Further investigations are thus needed to elicit a cause: MRI and magnetic resonance venogram are appropriate to exclude an intracranial venous sinus thrombosis. Other investigations may include: thyroid function tests; auto-immune profile; immunoglobulins; rheumatoid factor; antineutrophil cytoplasmic antibody; angiotensin converting enzyme; CSF oligoclonal bands; Lyme disease and viral serology.

BIH is usually self limiting. Once the CSF pressure has been reduced, any offending drugs should be discontinued. For symptomatic control, intracranial pressure can be reduced by: daily lumbar puncture with CSF drainage, or large doses of acetazolamide +/− loop diuretic. The role of steroids is controversial. If symptoms are unremitting, or there is ongoing visual impairment, then a surgical lumbo-peritoneal shunt or optic nerve fenestration may be required, as infarction of the optic nerve can occur. Notable clinical features may include a sixth nerve palsy, and partial or complete monocular visual loss − the only serious neurologic sign. The normal blind spots are commonly enlarged.

CASE 8.13

A 9-year-old girl presented with a 2-week history of polyuria and polydipsia. She appeared well on admission and the only abnormality to find on examination was a smooth, non-tender goitre. Her blood sugar was 17 mmol/l and she was commenced on subcutaneous insulin. Her thyroid tests showed:

TSH 0.2 miu/l
Free T4 31.9 pmol/l
Free T3 10 pmol/l

a. What is the most likely cause of her thyroid problem?
SELECT *ONE* ANSWER ONLY
  i. Hashimoto's thyroiditis
 ii. Grave's disease
iii. Pendred's syndrome
 iv. De Quervain's thyroiditis
  v. Secondary hypothyroidism

b. What other autoimmune conditions may be associated with diabetes mellitus?
SELECT *THREE* ANSWERS ONLY
  i. Addison's disease
 ii. Gastric autoimmunity
iii. The polyglandular autoimmune syndromes
 iv. Dermatomyositis
  v. Autoimmune hepatitis
 vi. Systemic lupus erythematosus

ANSWERS TO CASE 8.13

a. i. Hashimoto's thyroiditis
b. i. Addison's disease
    ii. Gastric autoimmunity
    iii. The polyglandular autoimmune syndromes

Although she currently has biochemical hyperthyroidism, she is likely to become hypothyroid secondary to chronic thyroiditis. Autoimmune thyroid disease is the most common autoimmune disease occurring in families with IDDM, and Hashimoto's thyroiditis is the most common underlying diagnosis. Thyroid microsomal antibodies are present in about 20% of diabetic children less than 16 years of age. In antibody-positive subjects, approximately 7% will become hypothyroid; 1% will suffer from Grave's disease.

Associated autoimmune diseases are relatively common in children with IDDM, particularly in children who have HLA-DR3. Some conditions may precede the onset of diabetes; others develop later. The following are associated autoimmune diseases:

- Hypothyroidism: 2-5% of children with IDDM
- Hyperthyroidism: 1% of children with IDDM
- Addison's disease: <1% but life-threatening (may reduce insulin requirement), diagnosis may be suspected when growth velocity falls off, or when an individual develops a marked sensitivity to insulin, with frequent episodes of hypoglycaemia, which often precedes classical markers of Addison's disease
- Coeliac disease, such as increased pigmentation or electrolyte disturbances
- Necrobiosis lipoidica: 1-2% of children with IDDM

Parietal cell antibodies (PCA) are present in approximately 10% of children with diabetes, but rarely progress to clinical disease. However, achlorhydria is not uncommon in PCA-positive diabetic children and may lead to iron deficiency.

Polyglandular autoimmune syndromes present in three types:

Type I: rare and presents in childhood, it usually comprises mucocutaneous candidiasis, hypoparathyroidism and primary adrenal insufficiency.

Type II: most common and defined as primary adrenal insufficiency with either autoimmune thyroid disease or type I diabetes mellitus occurring in the same individual (primary hypogonadism, myasthenia gravis, and coeliac disease also occur).

Type III: the co-occurrence of autoimmune thyroid disease with two other autoimmune disorders, including IDDM (type I), pernicious anaemia or a non-endocrine, organ-specific, autoimmune disorder in the absence of Addison's disease.

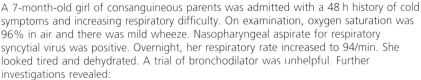
A 7-month-old girl of consanguineous parents was admitted with a 48 h history of cold symptoms and increasing respiratory difficulty. On examination, oxygen saturation was 96% in air and there was mild wheeze. Nasopharyngeal aspirate for respiratory syncytial virus was positive. Overnight, her respiratory rate increased to 94/min. She looked tired and dehydrated. A trial of bronchodilator was unhelpful. Further investigations revealed:

Hb 11.1 g/dl
WBC 38.3 × 10⁹/l (neutrophils 20.8 × 10⁹/l, lymphocytes 12.3 × 10⁹/l)

Platelets 741 × 10⁹/l
CXR mild hyperinflation
Capillary blood gas (pH 6.932, pO₂ 6.81 kPa, pCO₂ 2.01 kPa, standard bicarbonate 3.0 mmol/l, base excess −28.4)
Serum ammonia 51 μmol/l (normal range 21-47 μmol/l)
Serum lactate 11.5 mmol/l (normal range 1.0-1.8 mmol/l)
Blood glucose 2.2 mmol/l.

a. What is the most likely cause of this child's deterioration?
SELECT *ONE* ANSWER
  i. Hypoglycaemia
 ii. Fulminant lactic acidosis
iii. Severe hypocarbia
 iv. Septic shock
  v. Pulmonary hypertension

b. What further steps should be taken to manage her?
SELECT *TWO* ANSWERS
   i. Intubation and ventilation to help correct acidosis
  ii. i.v. sodium benzoate
 iii. 20 ml/kg bolus of 10% dextrose
  iv. Total parenteral nutrition
   v. i.v. sodium bicarbonate to correct acidosis
  vi. Bolus of 50% dextrose
 vii. Broad-spectrum antibiotics

ANSWERS TO CASE 8.14

a. ii. Fulminant lactic acidosis
b. v. i.v.sodium bicarbonate to correct acidosis
   vii. Broad-spectrum antibiotics

This child has developed fulminant lactic acidosis, secondary to acute metabolic decompensation of an underlying metabolic disorder. Management involves high-dependency care, and liaison with a specialist metabolic unit for advice on further investigations and management.

The metabolic acidosis should be corrected by an infusion of i.v. sodium bicarbonate.

Fluids should be 5% dextrose (there is no need for a bolus here and 10% dextrose is used as a bolus for hypoglycaemia). Protein should be excluded from the fluids since it would increase the metabolic acidosis. Broad-spectrum antibiotics should be given to cover the possibility of infection.

Metabolic disease should always be considered in unusual presentations. The main pointers towards a metabolic disorder are severe metabolic acidosis, lactic acidosis, hypoglycaemia, a raised ammonia level and episodes precipitated by an intercurrent infection. It is unlikely to be a urea cycle disorder as blood ammonia was only slightly raised, the lactic acidosis was severe and the child was not showing any neurological symptoms.

Organic acidaemias can present with raised blood ammonia and severe metabolic acidosis because of accumulation of organic acids in body fluids, but in this child, blood ammonia was only slightly raised. There appears to be a defect in intermediary carbohydrate metabolism associated with lactic acidosis. Indeed, this child was found to have fructose-1,6-diphosphate deficiency, which was confirmed on white cells enzyme studies. Fructose-1,6-diphosphate enzyme is one of the enzymes in the pathway of gluconeogenesis, and is also needed for the conversion of fructose to glucose. Symptoms may be precipitated by starvation, intake of fructose or sucrose and intercurrent illnesses.

CASE 8.15

A female infant was born at 26 weeks' gestation by spontaneous vertex delivery. Her mother was para 2 + 0 and previously well; she had received i.m. betamethasone 4 h prior to delivery. The baby received two doses of surfactant within 12 h of birth, and completed 48 h of antibiotics which were stopped when the blood cultures and surface swabs, taken shortly after birth, were negative for infection. She is now 8 days old, has been ventilated since birth and is, at present, on half-enteral and half-parenteral feeding.

Her present ventilator settings are peak inspiratory pressure of 20 cm of water, end expiratory pressure of 4 cm of water, inspiratory time of 0.42 s and inspired oxygen concentration of 40%. The ventilator is set to patient-triggered ventilation mode.

You are called when there has been a sudden deterioration in oxygen saturations and a drop in the heart rate.

On examination her oxygen saturation is 54%, heart rate 74 bpm and capillary refill time <2 s measured over the sternum. There is poor chest movement with poor air entry bilaterally. Her heart sounds are normal and there is no murmur.

What are the most likely causes?

SELECT *THREE* ANSWERS ONLY
  i. Blocked endotracheal tube
 ii. Tension pneumothorax
iii. Air trapping
 iv. Pulmonary hypertension with right to left shunting
  v. Duct-dependent congenital heart disease
 vi. Pneumonia
vii. Pulmonary haemorrhage
viii. Ventilator failure

ANSWERS TO CASE 8.15

   i. Blocked endotracheal tube
   ii. Tension pneumothorax,
 viii. Ventilator failure

Any acute deterioration in a baby on a ventilator must raise the possibility of a mechanical failure, either with the ventilator itself, which should be checked thoroughly, or by a blocked or dislodged endotracheal tube, which would show reduced chest movement, or a pneumothorax. Other causes of acute deterioration, e.g. intraventricular haemorrhage or sepsis, would not result in poor chest movement as a new finding. Pulmonary haemorrhage is usually accompanied by fresh blood from the endotracheal tube.

Examination with a cold light source would diagnose a pneumothorax, which can occur as a complication in any ventilated baby.

Immediate management in this case involves checking the tube position by auscultation over stomach as well as lung fields, suctioning of tube and changing the tube if it is blocked or dislodged, and decompression of a pneumothorax, if detected, by needle thoracocentesis in the second intercostal space. A definitive chest drain can then be inserted electively once the baby has been stabilised.

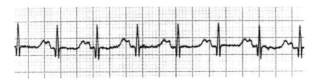

Fig 8.16

A previously well, term baby suffers a cardiac arrest on the postnatal ward on day 2 of life. Resuscitation efforts are successful.

a. What does her ECG show?
    SELECT *TWO* ANSWERS ONLY
    i. 1st degree heart block
    ii. P mitrale
    iii. Long QT interval
    iv. P wave occurring during repolarization phase
    v. Atrial flutter
    vi. Tachycardia

b. With what are these findings associated?
    SELECT *TWO* ANSWERS ONLY
    i. 22q11 deletion
    ii. Tricyclic antidepressants
    iii. Hypertrophic obstructive cardiomyopathy
    iv. Clindamycin
    v. Jervell–Lange–Nielson syndrome

ANSWERS TO CASE 8.16

a. iii. Long QT interval
   iv. P wave occurring during repolarization phase
b. ii. Tricyclic antidepressants

The ECG shows a long QT interval. The QT interval varies with heart rate, and thus the corrected QT interval (QTc) is calculated:

$$QTc = \frac{QT \text{ interval}}{\sqrt{R\text{-}R \text{ interval}}}$$

where QT = time (s) from beginning of Q wave to end of T wave. Normal value of QTc is <0.45 s.

Congenital long QT has two main variants: Romano–Ward, which is the more common type, and the Jervell–Lange–Nielson form, which may be due to a recessive gene and is associated with deafness.

The drug cisapride has been associated with prolonged QT interval, as have various other medications including some antibiotics and antifungals (e.g. erythromycin and fluconazole), terfenadine and tricyclic antidepressants.

Long-term oral beta-blockers decrease the risk of arrhythmias. Effectiveness is debatable, but in infants the incidence of arrhythmia in the first year of life is decreased from 50% to less than 10%.

Implantable defibrillators are effective but size limits their use to patients over 2 years old.

A 6-week-old girl is referred for investigation of prolonged jaundice and failure to thrive. On examination she is also noted to have a heart murmur in the pulmonary area and 3 cm hepatomegaly. Blood results show conjugated bilirubinaemia. Interestingly, her 5-year-old sister is noted to be short, has been requiring extra help in school and also has a heart murmur.

a. What would be the main investigations for the 6-week-old?
   SELECT *TWO* ANSWERS ONLY
   i. Stool for reducing substances
   ii. Thyroid function tests
   iii. Echocardiography
   iv. Liver isotope scan
   v. Direct Coombs' test

b. What is the likely diagnosis?
   SELECT *ONE* ANSWER ONLY
   i. Biliary atresia
   ii. Alagille syndrome
   iii. Gilbert's syndrome
   iv. α1-antitrypsin deficiency
   v. Congenital hypothyroidism

c. What is the inheritance of this condition?
   SELECT *ONE* ANSWER ONLY
   i. X-linked dominant
   ii. Autosomal dominant
   iii. Autosomal recessive
   iv. X-linked recessive
   v. Sporadic

ANSWERS TO CASE 8.17

a. iii. Echocardiography
   iv. Liver isotope scan
b. ii. Alagille syndrome
c. ii. Autosomal dominant

The baby should have a liver isotope excretion scan plus liver biopsy to exclude biliary atresia as this would require prompt operative management.

These sisters have Alagille syndrome (arteriohepatic dysplasia). Patients with this syndrome typically have chronic cholestasis, characteristic facies with a small pointed chin, vertebral arch defects, peripheral pulmonary artery hypoplasia or stenosis or other congenital heart disease, failure to thrive and mild to moderate learning difficulties.

Inheritance is autosomal dominant with variable expression. In this family the older sister had minimal liver involvement.

Ophthalmology examination to look for anterior chamber abnormalities (posterior embryotoxon), X-rays to look for abnormal vertebrae and blood for hypercholesterolaemia can help confirm the diagnosis.

CASE 8.18

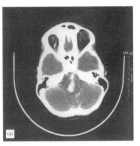 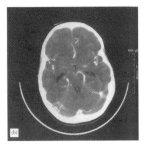 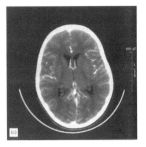

Fig 8.18

A 9-year-old boy presented to the A&E department at 02.00 h, with severe neck pain, vomiting and drowsiness. He was well on going to bed. There was a history of headaches over the last few months but no other relevant history. On examination, GCS was 13, there was neck stiffness but no rash or fever. There were no focal neurological signs. The fundi could not be visualised clearly. There were no other physical signs. The cranial CT scans are illustrated.

What does the cranial CT scan show?

SELECT *TWO* ANSWERS ONLY
  i. Mass lesion in foramen magnum
 ii. Intraventricular blood
iii. Subarachnoid haemorrhage
 iv. Space-occupying lesion right orbit
  v. Normal sized ventricles
 vi. Cerebral oedema

ANSWERS TO CASE 8.18

i. Mass lesion in foramen magnum

ii. Intraventricular blood

The history suggests several possible differential diagnoses: spontaneous subarachnoid haemorrhage, traumatic subdural or extradural haemorrhage, acutely raised intracranial pressure or meningitis.

Whatever the cause the initial management involves ABCD assessment. The conscious level and pupillary responses should be observed and assessed regularly. Blood glucose should be checked in any patient with a decreased conscious level. This patient needs an urgent CT scan, and neurosurgical and paediatric intensive care unit consultation is required early. In view of his reduced conscious level, he should not have a lumbar puncture.

The CT shows an extra-axial mass lesion in the anterior aspect of the foramen magnum extending up to the pons, displacing and compressing the medulla posteriorly to the left. There is intraventricular blood and early hydrocephalus. Both vertebral arteries are seen along with the mass lesion at the level of the foramen magnum. The lesion is likely to be an aneurysm arising from the vertebro-basilar junction projecting posteriorly. This patient presented with a very acute history compatible with intracranial haemorrhage. The headaches raised the possibility of a brain tumour or other space-occupying lesion. Infection was much less likely. CT scan showed a brain stem vascular malformation with haemorrhage, and blood in the subarachnoid and intraventricular spaces. Despite urgent neurosurgical referral, this patient deteriorated with further brain stem bleeding and died.

CASE 8.19

A 7-year-old girl was referred to the endocrine clinic having developed axillary and pubic hair over the last year. There was no breast development and she was premenarchal. More recently, she had developed an adult body odour. On examination she looked well and was normotensive. She had some short dark hairs over her mons pubis but no cliteromegaly and longer darker hairs in her axillae (Tanner stage 2).

What is the differential diagnosis?

SELECT *THREE* ANSWERS ONLY

   i. Premature adrenarche
  ii. Premature menarche
 iii. Premature thelarche
 iv. Congenital adrenal hyperplasia
  v. Precocious puberty
 vi. Constitutional precocious puberty
vii. Androgen-secreting tumour

ANSWERS TO CASE 8.19

i. Premature adrenarche
iv. Congenital adrenal hyperplasia
vii. Androgen-secreting tumour

The most likely diagnosis is premature adrenarche, but congenital adrenal hyperplasia (non-classical or simple virilising) and an androgen-secreting tumour of the adrenal glands or ovaries must be considered.

Adrenarche (with the isolated appearance of pubic hair) is puberty of the adrenal gland and is considered premature before the age of 8 years. It is characterised by greasy hair and skin, weight gain, slight pubic hair development and an adult body odour. The bone age may be slightly advanced but adrenarche has no effect on final height. The chief hormone produced is dehydroepiandrosterone sulphate (DHEAS); proposed aetiologies include a maturational increase in 17α-hydroxylase and 17,20-lyase enzymes and a reduction in 3β-hydroxysteroid dehydrogenase (3β-HSD). Although generally mild, the signs of adrenarche can be exaggerated and this can make it difficult to distinguish clinically from congenital adrenal hyperplasia (CAH) or an androgen-secreting tumour. Cliteromegaly often indicates a more serious cause of virilisation. CAH presents with rapid growth and virilisation with cliteromegaly, most commonly due to 21α-hydroxylase enzyme deficiency. Rather than presenting as a classical salt-wasting type, the differential diagnosis in this case would be a simple virilising or late onset/nonclassical congenital adrenal hyperplasia. 11β-hydroxylase deficiency is rare, presenting with virilisation and hypertension due to excess deoxycorticosterone levels. 3β-HSD deficiency is rare and presents with mild virilisation due to excess DHEAS levels.

Androgen-secreting tumours often have a shorter history and clinical signs progress rapidly. Girls with premature adrenarche may be at increased risk of developing polycystic ovarian syndrome. Investigations include:
- Biochemical investigations: basal androgens (testosterone, androstenedione, DHEAS), basal 17-OHP and urine steroid profile
- Radiological investigations: bone age and pelvic ultrasound scan
- Further investigations: in cases where it is difficult to distinguish between adrenarche and other causes of virilisation, one can consider a Synacthen test measuring cortisol and 17-OHP (in non-classical 21-hydroxylase deficiency CAH, basal 17-OHP may be normal but on Synacthen stimulation, the 17-OHP will show an exaggerated response) and a CT scan of the adrenal glands may be required if adrenal or ovarian tumours are suspected.

Chapter

A 3 h old baby, born at term in good condition after a normal pregnancy, was found on the postnatal ward to be intermittently jerking. On examination, he was profoundly floppy and unrousable. His blood sugar was 4.2 mmol/l. Arterial blood gas: pH 7.03, pCO_2 9.5 kPa, pO_2 5.1 kPa, HCO_3 19 mmol/l and BE −3.2. He was transferred to the neonatal unit and ventilated. Full septic and metabolic screens were performed.

There was no hepatomegaly. CXR was unremarkable. U&Es, LFTs, calcium and magnesium levels were normal, as were blood lactic acid and ammonia levels. With ventilation, his respiratory acidosis corrected rapidly. An EEG showed burst suppression.

The baby continued to fit despite treatment with phenobarbitone. He lost all respiratory drive, and became unresponsive to pain. Cultures of blood, urine and CSF were negative. The metabolic screen revealed an elevated glycine level in the CSF, and an increased CSF/plasma glycine ratio.

a. Suggest a diagnosis:
    SELECT *ONE* ANSWER ONLY
  i. OTC deficiency
  ii. Peroxisomal disorder
  iii. Non-ketotic hyperglycinaemia
  iv. MCAD deficiency
  v. Urea cycle disorder

b. What therapies may be used in the treatment of this condition?
    SELECT *TWO* ANSWERS ONLY
  i. Carnitine
  ii. Vitamin B12
  iii. Benzodiazepines
  iv. Forced alkaline diuresis
  v. Dextromethorphan (NMDA receptor blocker)
  vi. Sodium benzoate

ANSWERS TO CASE 9.1

a. iii. Non-ketotic hyperglycinaemia
b. v. Dextromethorphan
    vi. Sodium benzoate

This metabolic condition causes acute neurological distress, without hyperammonaemia, or metabolic acidosis, in the first hours of life. It is characterised by coma, hypotonia and myoclonic jerks. The inheritance is autosomal recessive, with the metabolic lesion being in the glycine cleavage system, a complex enzyme system with four enzyme components.

Other conditions such as sulphite oxidase deficiency and perioxisomal disorders can present in a similar way; however, they are associated with dysmorphism, and usually present later. The diagnosis of NKH relies on the demonstration of elevated glycine in the CSF, and especially an elevated CSF/plasma glycine ratio. An EEG usually always shows a burst suppression pattern.

Liaison with a neuro-metabolic specialist in a tertiary centre is essential. No consistent effective treatment is known. High levels of glycine cause overstimulation of the N-methyl-D-aspartate (NMDA) receptors in the brain. Dextromethorphan, an NMDA receptor blocker, has been used with variable success, as has sodium benzoate, which conjugates glycine. L-carnitine, which promotes glycine conjugation with benzoate, has also been tried.

Despite the above therapies, the prognosis is extremely poor. Most infants die in the neonatal period, and those that survive have severe mental retardation. Prenatal diagnosis is now available for affected families.

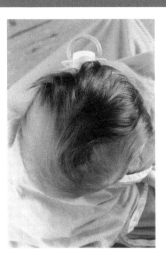

Fig 9.2

A 5-month-old baby is referred by the GP who is concerned about the head shape. The baby is thriving, there are no associated dysmorphic features, and the deformity is not progressing.

a. What is the diagnosis?
   SELECT *ONE* ANSWER ONLY
   i. Brachycephaly
   ii. Scaphocephaly
   iii. Hydrocephaly
   iv. Plagiocephaly

b. What investigation is needed?
   SELECT *ONE* ANSWER ONLY
   i. SXR
   ii. CT head
   iii. None
   iv. Cranial ultrasound scan

ANSWERS TO CASE 9.2

a. iv. Plagiocephaly
b. iii. None

This abnormal head shape resembling a parallelogram is known as plagiocephaly. The most common cause of this condition is due to postural factors, which result from external forces applied to the soft infant skull. Risk factors associated with plagiocephaly include:

Restrictive intrauterine environment – such as large baby, multiple pregnancies, small maternal pelvis, small or malformed uterus, etc.

Prematurity – this makes the already malleable cranium even more susceptible to the moulding forces

Back sleeping – following the "Back to Sleep" campaign to reduce the risk of sudden infant death syndrome, the number of infants presenting with plagiocephaly increased.

Detailed clinical examination is needed to rule out dysmorphic features associated with craniosynostosis. If the deformity is severe and progressive, or if associated with other dysmorphic features, SXR and CT scan should be undertaken to exclude craniosynostosis. Syndromes associated with craniosynostosis include Apert syndrome, Crouzon syndrome and Pfeiffer syndrome.

Management of simple plagiocephaly involves a conservative approach with reassurance. The deformity becomes less obvious with age and scalp hair growth.

CASE 9.3

A 10-year-old boy presented with a 24 h history of pyrexia, vomiting and tachypnoea. His parents reported that, over the past month, he had been losing weight despite eating well, and drinking more than usual. Otherwise he had been in very good health. On examination, he was thin, more than 5% dehydrated, with a sighing respiratory pattern.

Biochemistry: Na 148 mmol/l, K 4.1 mmol/l, urea 7.8 mmol/l, creatinine 67 µmol/l and bicarbonate 14 mmol/l.

a. Give three further initial relevant investigations:
   SELECT *THREE* ANSWERS ONLY
   i. Blood glucose
   ii. Urinalysis
   iii. FBC
   iv. Bone marrow aspiration
   v. CXR
   vi. Echocardiogram
   vii. Short synacthen test
   viii. Blood gas

His condition improved with appropriate treatment, and he was discharged home 2 days later on regular medication. Two months later, he awoke with a moderate right hemiparesis which resolved completely over the next 10 h.

b. What complication of his treatment is likely to have occurred?
   SELECT THE *BEST* ANSWER
   i. Microembolic cerebrovascular accident
   ii. Todd's paresis
   iii. Fat embolus
   iv. Intracerebral haemorrhage
   v. Sagittal venous thrombosis

ANSWERS TO CASE 9.3

a.   i. Blood glucose
    ii. Urinalysis
  viii. Blood gas
b. ii. Todd's paresis

This child initially presented in diabetic ketoacidosis. The history of weight loss, poly-dipsia, and polyuria in a previously well child is typical. Hypoglycaemia is a complica-tion of treatment, and in this case was significant enough to precipitate a seizure, complicated by a Todd's palsy. Complete resolution of the neurological deficit is expected.

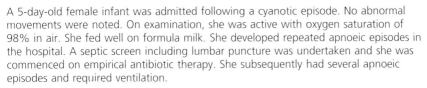
A 5-day-old female infant was admitted following a cyanotic episode. No abnormal movements were noted. On examination, she was active with oxygen saturation of 98% in air. She fed well on formula milk. She developed repeated apnoeic episodes in the hospital. A septic screen including lumbar puncture was undertaken and she was commenced on empirical antibiotic therapy. She subsequently had several apnoeic episodes and required ventilation.

On day 2 of mechanical ventilation, she was on pressures of 14/3.5, a rate of 30/min and 30% FiO2.

Blood gas analysis showed:
  pH 7.42
  pCO_2 5.4 kPa
  pO_2 8.1 kPa
  BE 6.3

The results of other investigations:
  Blood, urine and CSF cultures were negative
  CXR was normal
  ECG was normal
  Serum ammonia and lactate levels were normal

On day 5, she was extubated and commenced on feeds. She again developed apnoeic episodes.

a. What is the most likely diagnosis?
  SELECT *ONE* ANSWER ONLY
  i. Subclinical seizures
  ii. Gastroesophageal reflux
  iii. H-type tracheo-oesophageal fistula
  iv. Bulbar palsy with swallowing incoordination
  v. Patent ductus arteriosus

b. What investigation is most useful to confirm this diagnosis?
  SELECT *ONE* ANSWER ONLY
  i. EEG
  ii. Prone oesophagram
  iii. pH study
  iv. Echocardiogram
  v. Upper gastrointestinal contrast study

ANSWERS TO CASE 9.4

a. ii. Gastroesophageal reflux
b. iii. pH study

Gastro-oesophageal reflux is the most likely cause. In this case it was secondary to congenital hypertrophic pyloric stenosis. This condition occurs more frequently in male infants. This infant had a family history of congenital pyloric stenosis.

Investigations should include an oesophageal pH study and an upper GI contrast, and a test to exclude pyloric stenosis if necessary.

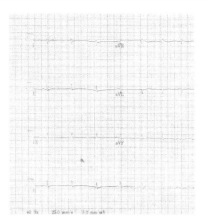

Fig 9.5

A 15-year-old boy was referred by his GP with possible pneumonia. He had a 2 week history of cough and acute onset of chest pain made worse by deep breathing. There was no history of vomiting, haemoptysis or injury. Past history was unremarkable and he was on pizotifen for headaches. Initial examination revealed the following:
Temperature 37.7°C
Oxygen saturation 99% in air
Respiratory rate 22/min
Blood pressure 110/66 mmHg

There was no chest wall tenderness, no wheeze or crackles, and the abdomen was soft with no evidence of hepatosplenomegaly. An ECG (see Fig. 9.5) and CXR were carried out.

The haematological and biochemical investigations were as follows:
Hb 18.6 g/dl
WBC 9.6 (neutrophils 6.4, lymphocytes 1.8)
platelets 376
ESR 31
CRP 104
ALP 187
Albumin 41
Corrected Ca 2.44

An echocardiogram confirmed a small pericardial effusion and normal ventricles. The chest X-ray was reported by the radiologist as "marked widening of the mediastinum suggestive of extensive mediastinal lymphadenopathy; the lungs appear clear".

What is your differential diagnosis?

SELECT *THREE* ANSWERS ONLY
i. Amyloidosis
ii. Tuberculosis
iii. Cardiomyopathy
iv. Glycogen storage disease
v. Sarcoidosois
vi. Leukaemia
vii. Mucopolysaccharidosis type IV
viii. Carcinoma of the bronchus

ANSWERS TO CASE 9.5

ii. Tuberculosis
v. Sarcoidosis
vi. Leukaemia

Differential diagnoses should include malignancy, lymphoma, leukaemia, tuberculosis, and sarcoidoses.

Further investigations needed are a repeat FBC and blood film, lactate dehydrogenase, a Mantoux test and a CT scan of chest and abdomen.

The ECG shows low voltage in all leads suggestive of pericarditis. Bacterial infection accounts for 1-8% of cases and causes purulent pericarditis. These develop from direct pulmonary extension, haematogenous spread, myocardial abscess/endocarditis, penetrating injury to chest wall from either trauma or surgery, or a subdiaphragmatic suppurative lesion. Organisms isolated include Gram-positive species such as *Streptococcus pneumoniae*, other Streptococcus species and Staphylococcus, and Gram-negative species, including *Proteus, E. coli, Pseudomonas, Klebsiella, Salmonella, Shigella, Neisseria meningitidis and Haemophilus influenzae*. Less common organisms include *Legionella, Nocardia, Actinobacillus, Rickettsia* and *Lyme borreliosis (Borrelia burgdorferi)*. Tuberculosis accounts for 4% of cases and viral infections account for 1-10% of cases. Causative viruses include coxsackie B, echovirus, adenoviruses, influenza A and B viruses, enterovirus, mumps virus, EBV, HIV, HSV1, varicella zoster virus, measles virus, parainfluenza 2 virus and respiratory syncytial virus. Other causes include renal failure, autoimmune disease, rheumatic fever and malignancy. The ECG is classically low voltage in all leads. Four stages of ECG changes are described in acute pericarditis; however, many patients will not exhibit all four stages.

The stages are as follows:
1. ST segment elevation and PR segment may be depressed.
2. ST segment is still elevated but returning to baseline with decreased T-wave amplitude. PR segment is depressed.
3. ST segment returns to normal with T-wave inversion (may be incomplete in some cases).
4. ECG normalisation occurs. T-wave changes may persist and do not necessarily indicate active disease.

A 9-year-old girl presented to the outpatient clinic with a history of becoming increasingly clumsy. She had been diagnosed as dyspraxic 2 years previously.

Her parents described her as always having been clumsy. They noted her balance was becoming worse over the previous 6-12 months. She was increasingly prone to falls and found walking in a straight line very difficult. She could not manage zips or buttons, and her writing was large, slow and difficult to read.

Examination revealed a pleasant, co-operative 9 year old girl. She had a 1 cm × 2 cm café au lait patch on her left anterior chest wall. She had a mild thoracic scoliosis. There was no pes cavus or clawing of her toes. General examination was otherwise unremarkable. Neurological examination revealed normal cranial nerve function. There was normal tone and power in the upper limbs, and reflexes were present, although difficult to elicit. She displayed bilateral finger nose ataxia.

Lower-limb assessment revealed normal power with slight reduction in tone. Her knee and ankle jerks were absent bilaterally. Plantars were extensor and she had reduced proprioception. Her gait was ataxic with poor balance. Romberg's sign was positive.

What is the likely diagnosis?

SELECT *ONE* ANSWER ONLY

   i. Cerebellar syndrome
  ii. Hereditary sensori-motor neuropathy
 iii. Friedrich's ataxia
 iv. Type II neurofibromatosis
  v. Refsum's disease
 vi. Kugelberg–Welander disease

ANSWER TO CASE 9.6

iii. Friedrich's ataxia

Early-onset ataxia sharing cerebellar and sensory elements, areflexia and scoliosis is very suggestive of Friedrich's ataxia, the most likely diagnosis in this case. Investigations include MRI brain scan, spine X-ray, ECG/echocardiogram, DNA for frataxin mutation and nerve conduction studies.

The onset of Friedrich's ataxia is between 2 and 16 years of age. It is autosomal recessive with an incidence of approximately one in 50 000. The initial feature is ataxia or clumsiness of gait in 95% of cases and scoliosis in 5%. Prognosis is poor with steady deterioration. Most patients are wheelchair dependent within 20 years of onset. All tendon reflexes are absent in 75% of children. Ninety per cent of patients have extensor plantar responses. Scoliosis develops in 80% of cases. Fifty-five percent of patients develop pes cavus, and 40% develop a cardiomyopathy. Treatment is supportive.

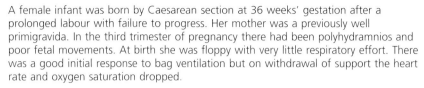

CASE 9.7

A female infant was born by Caesarean section at 36 weeks' gestation after a prolonged labour with failure to progress. Her mother was a previously well primigravida. In the third trimester of pregnancy there had been polyhydramnios and poor fetal movements. At birth she was floppy with very little respiratory effort. There was a good initial response to bag ventilation but on withdrawal of support the heart rate and oxygen saturation dropped.

On examination she was not moving, was hypotonic and had a poor suck. She also had bilateral talipes. She needed a gradual increase in ventilation pressures over the first 24 h. The CXR revealed hypoplastic lungs.

a. What is the most likely diagnosis?
SELECT *ONE* ANSWER ONLY
   i. Congenital hypothyroidism
  ii. Werndig–Hoffman disease
 iii. Congenital myotonic dystrophy
  iv. Congenital myasthenia gravis
   v. Prader–Willi syndrome
  vi. SMA type I
 vii. Congenital central hypoventilation syndrome

b. What investigation would you need to carry out to confirm your diagnosis?
SELECT *ONE* ANSWER ONLY
   i. Genetic studies
  ii. Muscle biopsy
 iii. Thyroid function tests
  iv. Tensilon test
   v. ECG

PASS

Questions and Answers for the New Format Exam

ANSWERS TO CASE 9.7

a. iii. Congenital myotonic dystrophy
b. i. Genetic studies

Congenital myotonic dystrophy (CMD) is the severest form of myotonic dystrophy (MD). In CMD, inheritance (autosomal dominant) appears to be almost exclusively from the mother. The diagnosis of myotonic dystrophy can be confirmed by looking for gene defect in chromosome 19.

The severity of disease is related to the number of repeats within the abnormal gene. Ventilation may be required for several weeks or even months but there may be a general improvement in muscle function after 3-4 months and if the neonatal period is survived, then the child will progress in a similar way to classic MD. Complications include mental retardation, learning difficulties, cataracts, hearing problems, cardiac arrhythmias and chronic constipation.

Other myopathies could present in a similar way but CMD is by far the most common. A pregnancy with an affected fetus is often complicated by polyhydramnios, and labour is likely to be prolonged because the mother is affected. Examination of the mother may aid the diagnosis – looking for myopathic facies and myotonia demonstrated by inability to relax firm hand grip (e.g. following hand shake).

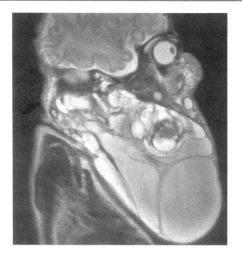

Fig 9.8

An antenatal ultrasound scan at 22 weeks' gestation revealed a large lesion in the neck of a female fetus. A postnatal T2-weighted MRI is shown.

a. In the antenatal period, which is the most important fetal investigation?
SELECT *ONE* ANSWER ONLY
 i. Nuchal thickness
 ii. Karyotype
 iii. Rhesus status
 iv. α-fetoprotein
 v. Fetal echocardiogram

b. What problem associated with this condition contributes to significant mortality?
SELECT *ONE* ANSWER ONLY
 i. Congenital heart disease
 ii. Hydronephrosis
 iii. Pulmonary hypoplasia
 iv. Hydrops fetalis
 v. Haemolytic disease of the newborn

ANSWERS TO CASE 9.8

a. ii. Karyotype
b. iv. Hydrops fetalis

This MRI shows a cystic hygroma (cystic lymphangioma). These occur with an incidence of approximately 1/6000 pregnancies. On ultrasound and MRI, they appear as complex multiloculated cystic masses, not infrequently having echogenic areas with haemorrhage. Nearly 80% of cystic hygromas involve the neck and frequently involve the floor of the mouth.

Antenatally, fetal karyotyping is necessary since about two-thirds of infants with an antenatal diagnosis of cystic hygroma will have an abnormal karyotype: 42% have XO (Turner's syndrome) and 18% have trisomies (of chromosomes 21, 18 and 13).

Cystic hygromas are associated with hydrops fetalis. Fetal death is a frequent outcome if hydrops is present. If the pregnancy continues, obstructed or complicated labour and delivery can occur. It is unusual for even very extensive lesions to interfere with swallowing in utero, leading to polyhydramnios. Other structural lesions may coexist, particularly in infants with an abnormal karyotype.

Very large masses such as this one may cause life-threatening airway compression. The immediate management is basic life support (ABC), first maintaining a stable patent airway. With an abnormality this size one must liaise antenatally with senior ENT surgeons, paediatric surgeons and anaesthetists. They may be required at delivery to stabilise the patient's airway.

Ex-utero intrapartum treatment (EXIT) has been described, the basic principle being the maintenance of intrapartum uteroplacental support while surgery is performed.

Definitive treatment consists of surgery. Complete excision is often not possible because these lesions often infiltrate deep structures with little regard for tissue boundaries. There is a high recurrence rate after excision. The other treatment option is the use of sclerosants. In particular, OK-432 (a lyophylized mixture of Streptococcus pyogenes) has been used successfully in several published cases.

CASE 9.9

A 4-year-old girl had DTP, Hib and oral polio at 2, 3 and 4 months of age. She is generally well, but had a febrile convulsion 10 days after her MMR at 18 months. Her 2-year-old brother is receiving chemotherapy for acute lymphoblastic leukaemia.

What immunisations, if any, should she not be given?

SELECT *ONE* ANSWER ONLY

i. Diphtheria, tetanus and pertussis booster
ii. Meningococcal C vaccine
iii. MMR
iv. Inactivated oral polio
v. i.m. polio
vi. None

ANSWER TO CASE 9.9

i. Diphtheria, tetanus and pertussis booster

Diphtheria and tetanus booster, meningococcal C vaccine, MMR with advice regarding temperature management, and inactivated polio (oral or intramuscular) in view of her immunocompromised sibling can all be given. Oral polio vaccine, which is a live vaccine and may be excreted in the stool, should not be given to immunosuppressed children, their siblings or other household contacts. Inactivated polio vaccine should be given instead.

A febrile convulsion is not a contraindication to further immunisations, but it is very important to watch the child closely for signs of fever. At the first observation of a rising temperature, paracetamol should be given 4-6 h.

Pertussis is not part of the pre-school booster schedule – it should be just diphtheria and tetanus.

CASE 9.10

A 23-month-old girl had been restless and crying overnight, with a fever, cough and hoarse voice. Next morning while awaiting a consultation with her family doctor, she had a generalised seizure in the waiting room. She was given rectal diazepam, she stopped fitting and was transferred by ambulance for evaluation in hospital. On arrival she was "post-ictal", had a temperature of 39.5°C, pulse rate of 90 bpm, respiratory rate of 25/min, and SaO_2 of 98% in room air. She was pale and hypotonic, with small pupils. The triage nurse checked her blood glucose using a blood glucose meter. The result was 0.9 mmol/l. A catheter urine sample was negative for standard dipstick parameters except +ve ketones.

Give three possible underlying diagnoses

SELECT *THREE* ANSWERS ONLY

   i. Organic acidurias
  ii. Alcohol ingestion
 iii. Beckwith–Wiedemann syndrome
 iv. Febrile convulsion
  v. Medium chain acyl CoA dehydrogenase deficiency
 vi. Diabetic ketoacidosis
vii. Paracetamol overdose

ANSWERS TO CASE 9.10

  i. Organic acidurias
  ii. Alcohol ingestion
  v. Medium chain acyl CoA dehydrogenase deficiency

After ABCs (airway, breathing, circulation), initial management of this child involves reversal of the hypoglycaemia. After gaining i.v. or intraosseous access, you need to administer a bolus of 10% dextrose followed by an infusion. If possible, take blood samples for later analysis before injecting the dextrose (see below). Relatively common causes of hypoglycaemia in this age group are ketotic hypoglycaemia and ingestion of alcohol or oral hypoglycaemic agents. Rare causes vary from hormone insufficiency (e.g. cortisol), liver disorders with hepatocellular failure, to a large range of inborn errors of gluconeogenesis, fatty acid oxidation disorders, ketolytic defects and organic acidurias. A systematic approach is required to ensure that no possibilities are overlooked. Hypoglycaemia should be confirmed by formal laboratory analysis. Investigations should include analysis for inborn errors (free fatty acids, plasma lactate, amino acids, −OH butyrate, cortisol and insulin).

This child was suffering from medium chain acyl CoA dehydrogenase (MCAD) deficiency. This autosomal recessive disorder of β-oxidation of fatty acids, generally presents clinically between the second month and second year of life, often triggered by minor illness. Hypoglycaemia occurs from an inability to oxidize fatty acids to ketones when glucose requirements cannot be met by gluconeogenesis. The combination of hypoglycaemia and cerebral oedema secondary to the toxic effects of fatty acid derivatives has a major impact on brain function and underlies the mortality – up to 20% at initial presentation. Initial laboratory examination of blood may reveal hypoglycaemia, mild metabolic acidosis, hyperammonaemia and high uric acid levels. Liver function may also be deranged. Examination of the urine often shows inappropriately low or absent ketones. Biochemical testing of blood and urine for carnitine, acylcarnitines, acylglycines and organic acids is diagnostic for the disorder.

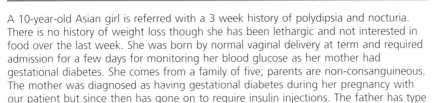

CASE 9.11

A 10-year-old Asian girl is referred with a 3 week history of polydipsia and nocturia. There is no history of weight loss though she has been lethargic and not interested in food over the last week. She was born by normal vaginal delivery at term and required admission for a few days for monitoring her blood glucose as her mother had gestational diabetes. She comes from a family of five; parents are non-consanguineous. The mother was diagnosed as having gestational diabetes during her pregnancy with our patient but since then has gone on to require insulin injections. The father has type 2 diabetes. The maternal grandparents died young, both had type 2 diabetes.

On examination her weight is > 99.6th centile and height is on the 98th centile. Her blood glucose on testing was 12.1.

What is her most likely diagnosis?

SELECT *ONE* ANSWER ONY
  i. Nephrogenic diabetes insipidus
  ii. Juvenile type 1 diabetes
  iii. Type 2 diabetes mellitus
  iv. Insulin dependent diabetes mellitus
  v. Cranial diabetes insipidus

ANSWER TO CASE 9.11

iii. Type 2 diabetes mellitus

Features that might give a clue to the diagnosis include obesity, acanthosis nigricans, and a family history of type 2 diabetes.

Conventional treatment of patients with type 2 diabetes usually begins with recommendations for life style changes (i.e. diet and physical activity) often in parallel with monotherapy with an oral agent such as metformin or gliclazide. If initial approaches fail, then a multidrug regimen, possibly including insulin, is prescribed. There may be a role for glitazone treatment in the paediatric age range, but this remains to be clarified. However, with the increasing recognition of the progressive nature of the disease and the high risk of micro- and macrovascular complications, it is recommended to treat it more aggressively to achieve glycaemic control.

Acanthosis nigricans is asymptomatic, brown-black, with a velvety texture. Pedunculated skin tags are often present. The most common sites are the axillae, neck, and groin. Its presence is associated with insulin resistance.

Recently, the number of type 2 cases has risen alarmingly in some parts of the world. In the Southern United States, type 2 diabetes accounts for over 30% of new cases of diabetes in childhood. There is some evidence of a similar increase in numbers in the UK. Most cases in the UK appear in the Asian subpopulation, although some Caucasian children may also be affected. Type 2 diabetes is characterised by both insulin resistance and deficient insulin secretion. Increasing obesity globally may be largely responsible for this increase. Treatment of these patients is complex because of the progressive nature of the disease and the multifaceted physiological defects. It can take years for subclinical hyperglycaemia to present as a symptomatic disease.

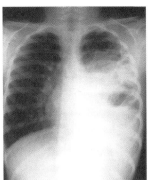

Fig 9.12.A

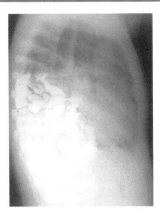

Fig 9.12.B

An 8-year-old boy who had been previously fit and well, was admitted with a rash and a dry cough. For 2 days he had eaten very little, and on admission he was apyrexial but sleepy. On examination, his respiratory rate was 30/min, with no recessions. He had decreased air entry over the left chest with some basal crackles. He also had a fading chickenpox rash over his trunk. A CXR was taken (see Fig. 9.12.A).

He improved over the next 24 h with i.v. antibiotics. It was noted that he had a history of constipation as an infant. On further examination 72 h after his admission, a contrast study was carried out (see Fig. 9.12.B).

What diagnosis does this contrast study confirm?

SELECT *ONE* ANSWER ONLY
   i. Left-sided hiatus hernia
   ii. Left lower lobe pneumonia with pneumatocoeles
   iii. Left-sided diaphragmatic hernia
   iv. Congenital eventration of the diaphragm
   v. Left-sided loculated empyema
   vi. Left pulmonary hypoplasia
   vii. Left-sided cystic adenomatoid malformation of the lung

ANSWER TO CASE 9.12

iii. Left-sided diaphragmatic hernia

Differential diagnoses from the X-ray alone include left lower lobe pneumonia, left-sided cystic congenital anomaly of the lung and a left-sided diaphragmatic hernia.

A barium meal examination shows contrast in the left thoracic cavity in loops of small bowel, confirming the diagnosis of diaphragmatic hernia.

Late presentation of congenital diaphragmatic hernia is rare. It is important to recognise, as, with appropriate treatment, all such children have a normal life expectancy. At any age, cystic lesions or masses in the lower lung fields should suggest the possibility of congenital diaphragmatic hernia.

An 11-year-old girl presents with a 4-week history of abnormal movements and difficulty walking. The school had noticed that her hand-writing had progressively deteriorated and she has difficulties with daily activities such as dressing and using cutlery. She has mild slurring of speech. The movements disappear during sleep. There are no other symptoms of note and no recent history of fever, rash or upper respiratory tract infection. Antenatal history and delivery were unremarkable. She has previously been healthy, takes no medication and her siblings are well. There is no family history of movement disorder or significant illness. On examination, she was alert, active and afebrile. She was normotensive. General examination was unremarkable. There was no organomegaly on abdominal examination. Fundoscopy showed normal appearances and cranial nerve examination was normal. She had bilateral choreiform movements in her hands on extension and pronation, and a positive "milkmaid sign". Choreiform movements of the tongue were also seen on attempted protrusion. Bulk and power were normal in all limbs but tone was slightly decreased.

What is the most likely diagnosis?

SELECT *ONE* ANSWER ONLY

   i. Posterior fossa tumour
  ii. Sydenham's chorea
 iii. Huntington's disease
 iv. Lesch–Nyhan syndrome
  v. Parkinson's disease
 vi. Pesticide poisoning

ANSWER TO CASE 9.13

ii. Sydenham's chorea

Sydenham's chorea is rare but the most likely diagnosis in the absence of clinical features to suggest alternative conditions.

Investigations should include:
- MRI brain, to exclude space-occupying lesion
- throat swab
- ASO and anti-Dnase B titre to look for supportive evidence of streptococcal infection
- ECG and echocardiogram to look for rheumatic carditis
- antinuclear antibody and ESR to exclude connective tissue disease
- thyroid function tests, PTH, U&E and bone profile should be checked, since hyperthyroidism, hypoparathyroidism and Addison's disease can present with chorea
- LFTs, serum copper and caeruloplasmin, amino acid screen, organic acid screen and lysosomal enzymes should also be checked

This list is by no means exhaustive as the conditions associated with chorea are protean. A toxicology screen should be considered in a child presenting acutely. Although there is no family history of Huntington's disease, DNA analysis for this disorder should be considered if other tests are inconclusive.

Haloperidol and diazepam may be used in the management of Sydenham's chorea. Secondary prophylaxis with penicillin V should be given until adulthood.

Jones' criteria for diagnosis of acute rheumatic fever

Two major versus one major and two minor criteria with evidence of a recent streptococcal infection.

Major criteria
- Carditis: 50% of patients with ARF and always associated with a murmur of valvulitis
- Polyarthritis: 70% of patients and manifested by a migratory arthritis of major joints
- Sydenham's chorea: 15% of patients and manifested by abnormal behaviour and/or involuntary, purposeless movements
- Erythema marginatum: 10% of patients and is an evanescent, pink rash with serpiginous borders
- Subcutaneous nodules: 2-10% of patients and manifested by painless nodules over extensor surfaces of large joints, the occiput, and/or vertebral processes

Minor criteria
- Arthralgia: can only be considered in the absence of arthritis
- Fever
- Elevated acute phase reactants: ESR, C-reactive protein
- Prolongation of the PR interval on ECG

Exceptions to the Jones' criteria include:

Sydenham chorea alone or indolent carditis alone (each of which may appear late, and therefore, may not be associated with supporting evidence of a recent streptococcal pharyngitis)

Patients with a previous diagnosis of ARF who have a recurrence may not fulfil the Jones' criteria due to the subtle presentation

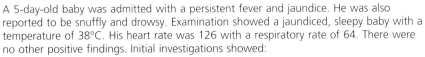

CASE 9.14

A 5-day-old baby was admitted with a persistent fever and jaundice. He was also reported to be snuffly and drowsy. Examination showed a jaundiced, sleepy baby with a temperature of 38°C. His heart rate was 126 with a respiratory rate of 64. There were no other positive findings. Initial investigations showed:

Hb 15.3 g/dl
WCC 5.0 × 10⁹/l
Platelets 119 × 10⁹/l
Na 136 mmol/l
K 4.0 mmol/l
Creatinine 41 μmol/l
Glucose 5.4 mmol/l
CRP 64 mg/l
AST 636 IU/l.

A CXR was unremarkable and lumbar puncture showed WBC 3/mm³, RBC 35/mm³, protein 0.84 g/l and glucose 2.6 mmol/l.

Over the next 24 h he became more unwell with poor perfusion and marked respiratory distress eventually requiring ventilatory support. In the same period he also had an episode of right-sided twitching lasting 30 s. Repeat examination revealed an enlarged liver and further investigations showed deranged clotting and an AST of 1399 IU/l.

a. What medication would you have added in when the baby deteriorated?
   SELECT *ONE* ANSWER ONLY
   i. Steroids
   ii. Mannitol
   iii. Acyclovir
   iv. Nitric oxide

b. What non-haematological investigation would be most useful in initially confirming the diagnosis?
   SELECT *ONE* ANSWER ONLY
   i. Urine for virus particles
   ii. CT scan
   iii. EEG
   iv. Skin swabs for virology

ANSWERS TO CASE 9.14

a. iii. Acyclovir
b. iii. EEG

Neonatal sepsis should be the initial diagnosis at presentation, and should be managed with resuscitation, an infection screen and initiation of appropriate antibiotics and ongoing supportive care. The most likely organism implicated in this age group is Group B streptococcus.

The diagnosis of suspected HSV infection is suggested by the age at presentation, the deranged clotting and massively elevated AST and the presence of seizures. The baby was subsequently proven to have disseminated HSV infection. It is important to note, as in this case, that there may be no maternal history of herpes infection.

An EEG would help in making the diagnosis, which characteristically shows temporo-parietal high-voltage, low-frequency activity in the presence of HSV meningoencephalitis.

CASE 9.15

A 6-month-old girl was being investigated for failure to thrive and passing loose, fatty, bulky stools. On examination she was found to be small (weight <3rd centile, birth weight 50th centile) and had a florid eczematous rash. Her sweat chloride was normal, and FBC showed a mild pancytopenia including an absolute neutropenia. A bone marrow aspirate was therefore undertaken.

a. What is the most likely diagnosis?
   SELECT *ONE* ANSWER ONLY
   i. Acute lymphoblastic leukaemia
   ii. Wiskott–Aldrich syndrome
   iii. Schwachmann's syndrome
   iv. Cystic fibrosis
   v. Diamond–Blackfan syndrome

b. What complications is she at risk of developing?
   SELECT *TWO* ANSWERS ONLY
   i. Diabetes mellitus
   ii. Sepsis
   iii. Malignancy
   iv. Hypertension
   v. Allergic bronchopulmonary aspergillosis
   vi. Cirrhosis of the liver

ANSWERS TO CASE 9.15

a. iii. Schwachmann's syndrome
b. ii. Sepsis
   iii. Malignancy

Schwachmann's syndrome is an autosomal recessive condition, and is the second most common cause of exocrine pancreatic insufficiency in the UK after CF.

The diagnosis is generally made after a combination of neutropenia (can be cyclical), thrombocytopenia and pancreatic insufficiency is found. Bone marrow aspirate and liver biopsy can aid diagnosis.

Complications include severe sepsis secondary to neutropenia, requiring inpatient treatment with broad-spectrum antibiotics, skeletal abnormalities secondary to metaphyseal dysplasia, and there is a small risk of leukaemic transformation, thus annual surveillance screening is necessary with bone marrow aspiration to look for leukaemic transformation.

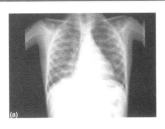 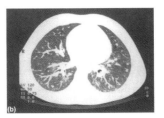

Fig 9.16

A 6-year-old girl presented a year ago with pallor (Hb 6.2 g/dl, MCV 69) and was found to be iron deficient. Five months later, she re-presented with intermittent cough productive of a small amount of blood. She had no history of fever. She was not breathless on exertion. On examination, she was mildly clubbed. On auscultation of her chest, there were bilateral basal crackles.

Investigations showed:
    Clotting normal
    U&E normal
    LFT normal
    Urinalysis – no blood or glucose; trace of protein
    Faecal occult blood positive.
Her CXR and CT scan are shown (Fig. 9.16.a, b)

a. What is the most likely diagnosis?
    SELECT *ONE* ANSWER ONLY
  i. Pulmonary haemosiderosis
  ii. Sickle cell disease
  iii. CF
  iv. TB

b. Select one other investigation to help confirm the diagnosis:
    SELECT *ONE* ANSWER ONLY
  i. Bronchoalveolar lavage microscopy
  ii. Pulmonary function tests
  iii. Sweat test
  iv. Mantoux test

ANSWERS TO CASE 9.16

a. i. Pulmonary haemosiderosis
b. i. Bronchoalveolar lavage microscopy

Pulmonary haemosiderosis is characterised by recurrent episodes of intra-alveolar haemorrhages, production of blood-stained sputum containing haemosiderin-laden macrophages and acute anaemia.

Sputum or bronchoalveolar lavage microscopy can be used to confirm the diagnosis; showing haemosiderin-laden macrophages. An open lung biopsy can also be performed; showing intra-alveolar haemorrhages and haemosiderin-laden macrophages within alveoli.

Aetiology

1. Primary: idiopathic
2. Secondary:
   i. cow's milk protein intolerance
   ii. Goodpasture's syndrome
   iii. heart disease, e.g. mitral stenosis
   iv. collagen vascular disease, e.g. polyarteritis, rheumatoid arthritis

Maintenance treatment includes inhaled steroids or low-dose, alternate-day, oral steroids. Azathioprine has been used. Some patients are able to discontinue treatment between acute episodes. Oral iron is given to correct anaemia.

The clinical course waxes and wanes in severity. Microscopic haemorrhages lead to chronic anaemia. Treatment of acute episodes consists of blood transfusion and i.v. hydrocortisone. Long-term prognosis is variable. Acute massive haemorrhages can be fatal.

An 8-month-old boy was admitted with a 4 hour history of breathing difficulty. On examination, he was apyrexial, he had a barking cough, inspiratory stridor and a respiratory rate of 35/min. He was treated with oral steroids. Over the next 48 h his condition fluctuated with periods of marked stridor and respiratory distress at night but improvement during the daytime. His condition worsened dramatically 72 h after admission; he appeared grey and sweaty with a high pyrexia, tachycardia and severe respiratory distress with oxygen saturations in the mid-80s.

What is the cause of his deterioration?

SELECT THE *MOST APPROPRIATE* ANSWER
  i. Epiglottitis
 ii. Septicaemic shock secondary to foreign body
iii. Bacterial tracheitis
 iv. Hypocalcaemia
  v. Anigoneurotic oedema

ANSWER TO CASE 9.17

iii. Bacterial tracheitis

The initial history here suggests viral laryngotracheobronchitis, i.e. croup. Bacterial tracheitis may occur as a secondary infection, usually in children less than 3 years old. Causative organisms include *Staphylococcus aureus, Haemophilus influenzae* and *Streptococcus pneumoniae*.

Management includes intubation and ventilation, frequent suctioning of the airway and appropriate antibiotics. At laryngoscopy mucosal swelling is seen at the level of the cricoid with thick, purulent secretions.

Complications include pneumonia, septicaemia, respiratory arrest, and subglottic stenosis.

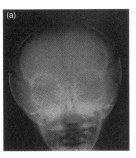 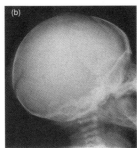 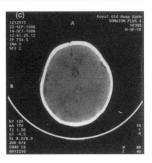

Fig 9.18

A 17-day-old baby was brought to the A&E department after his mother, who was carrying him in a baby sling, accidentally tripped and fell over. He had slipped from his baby sling on to the pavement hitting the front of his head, and had cried immediately. On examination, two large parietal swellings were noted, and neurological assessment was normal.

What do the SXR and CT scan show?

SELECT *TWO* ANSWERS ONLY

   i. SXR – normal
  ii. SXR – occipital fracture
 iii. SXR – bilateral parietal fractures
 iv. SXR – right temporal fracture
   v. CT – normal
 vi. CT – small right-sided subdural haemorrhage
 vii. CT – cerebral oedema with slit-like ventricles and midline shift
viii. CT – small right-sided extradural haemorrhage

ANSWERS TO CASE 9.18

iii. SXR – bilateral parietal fractures
vi. CT – small right-sided subdural haemorrhage

The SXR (AP view) demonstrates large bilateral parietal fractures. Figure (b) shows a lateral view of the skull, demonstrating fractures extending from the coronal sutures anteriorly, to the lamboidal sutures posteriorly. Figure (c) is a CT of the brain, showing a small right-sided subdural haemorrhage with no midline shift.

Further assessment should take the form of observation. In particular, the child's arousal state, pupil size and reactivity, heart rate, and blood pressure should be monitored at least half-hourly for 24 h, in order to detect any deterioration. The Glasgow neurological scale could not be applied directly in view of the child's age. Even scales specifically devised for children should be used cautiously in view of this boy's age and neurological immaturity. The subdural haemorrhage is small, so no surgical intervention is indicated. Should the child deteriorate and develop signs of raised intracranial pressure (drowsiness, vomiting, bradycardia and hypertension), a repeat CT scan is indicated to look for evidence of an extending lesion. The mother should be informed that the fractures will heal without intervention, and the subdural will gradually resolve. There should be no long-term sequelae but the child will be followed up.

One should consider the possibility of non-accidental injury, and a general examination should look at the general state of the child to ensure he is clean, thriving, and has not got any bruises of concern (although he will most certainly have bruises related to this injury). Ensure his frenulum is intact and there are no retinal haemorrhages. A skeletal survey and an ophthalmological examination should be arranged. Social services should be informed and a strategy meeting held. Liaison should also take place with the midwife and GP to ensure there are no concerns about this family.

CASE 9.19

1. Ostium secundum atrial septal defect
2. Ventricular septal defect
3. Transposition of the great arteries
4. Total anomalous pulmonary venous drainage
5. Atrioventricular septal defect
6. Patent ductus arteriosus
7. Pulmonary valve stenosis
8. Coarctation of the aorta
9. Tetralogy of Fallot
10. Hypoplastic left heart syndrome

For each of the following case scenarios select the most likely diagnosis from the list above:

a. An infant is seen for his 6-week check and found to have a loud ejection systolic murmur in the third left intercostal space and a single second heart sound on examination. There is no obvious cyanosis but a suggestion of mild desaturation. On the CXR there is a concavity on the left heart border and decreased pulmonary vascular markings.

b. An infant is found profoundly cyanosed and lethargic in his cot on day 2. On auscultation there is a soft systolic murmur heard inconsistently at the left sternal edge and a single second sound. The CXR shows a narrow upper mediastinum, hypertrophied right ventricle and increased pulmonary vascular markings. The ECG shows a normal neonatal pattern.

c. An 11-month-old girl presented to the local hospital with a 1 week history of cough, wheeziness and increasing lethargy. She was given bronchodilators but failed to respond. Her oxygen saturation on admission was only 70-80% despite 100% oxygen. She was intubated and ventilated and nitric oxide was given but without clinical improvement. On examination, she was cyanosed with a hyperactive praecordium. Her chest revealed scattered wheezes and crackles. There was a palpable liver of 2-3 cm. Her CXR showed a "cottage loaf" appearance.

a. 9. Tetralogy of Fallot

Fallot's tetralogy accounts for about 5% of congenital heart defects. The constituents of Fallot's tetralogy are: obstruction to right ventricular outflow tract, VSD, over-riding aorta and right ventricular hypertrophy. Children may be centrally pink in early infancy, but cyanosis is usually present by the end of the first year. There may be clubbing. Children have cyanotic "spells" due to decreased pulmonary blood flow which can occur during crying or exertion. To alleviate these spells, children may employ "squatting" which increases the systemic vascular resistance, reduces venous return from the legs and improves the pulmonary blood flow. Complications include cerebral thrombosis, cerebral abscess, bacterial endocarditis and a haemor-rhagic tendency.

b. 3. Transposition of the great arteries (TGA)

TGA constitutes about 5% of all congenital heart diseases and is the most common cyanotic heart disease present in the immediate postnatal period. It is slightly more common in males. In TGA, the normal serial circulation is changed to a parallel circulation resulting in complete separation of the systemic and pulmonary circuits. Hypoxaemic blood circulates in the body, whereas the hyperoxaemic blood circu-lates in the lungs. Defects such as a patent ductus arteriosus or atrial septal defect are crucial for mixing these two circuits and for survival. Because of this, infants usually present in the first few days of life when the PFO and PDA show signs of closure. Once the diagnosis is made, a prostin infusion should be commenced and transfer to a paediatric cardiac unit should be arranged. Often a Rashkind balloon septostomy is performed in infants with a small or closing atrial communication in order to improve mixing.

c. 4. Total anomalous pulmonary venous drainage (TAPVD)

In TAPVD, the pulmonary veins (PV) drain into the right atrium (RA) rather than into the left (LA). An atrial communication is essential for survival. TAPVD accounts for 1% of all congenital heart diseases and there is a marked male prepon-derance (4 : 1) in the infracardiac type. Four types are distinguished

Supracardiac: (50%) the common PV drains into the SVC via a vertical vein and the left innominate vein

Cardiac: (20%) the common PV drains into the coronary sinus or the PVs drain into the RA through four separate openings

Infracardiac: (20%) the common PV drains into the portal vein, ductus venosus, hepatic vein or the IVC

Mixed type: 10%: a combination of the other types

In the absence of PV obstruction, the child presents with mild cyanosis, growth retardation and heart failure; whereas in the case of PV obstruction, the presenta-tion is with severe cyanosis and respiratory distress in the neonatal period. The CXR showing the "snowman" or "cottage loaf" appearance is typical of supracardiac TAPVD. This appearance is usually only visible after 4 months of age.

Chapter 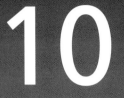 10

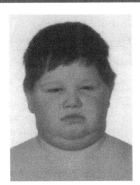

Fig 10.1.A

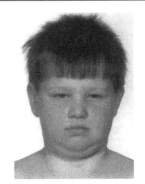

Fig 10.1.B

A12-year-old boy presented with a 3-year history of anxiety, school phobia and lack of energy during which he had gained excessive weight, despite a normal diet. Prior to this he had been fit and well with a normal birth history and no developmental concerns. His weight was 66.7 kg (above the 97th centile) and height 144.9 cm (25th centile). On examination he was obviously overweight, had coarse facies, very dry skin and absent ankle jerks (Fig. 10.1.A). There was a small palpable goitre and his pulse rate was 60 bpm. A bone age was delayed at 8.7 years. He was started on treatment and there was significant improvement in his symptoms and physical appearance (Fig. 10.1.B).

What is your clinical diagnosis?

SELECT *ONE* ANSWER ONLY

  i. Hypopituitarism
 ii. Craniopharyngioma
iii. Cushing's syndrome
 iv. Congenital hypothyroidism
  v. Acquired hypothyroidism
 vi. Euthyroidism

ANSWER TO CASE 10.1

v. Acquired hypothyroidism

The clinical diagnosis here is acquired hypothyroidism, which is most likely to be of autoimmune origin and also known as chronic lymphocytic thyroiditis. Both goitrous (Hashimoto's) and non-goitrous (primary myxoedema) forms are described. In about 30-40% of cases, there is often a strong family history of autoimmune thyroid disease. Presentation may be at any age but is more common during adolescence and is more common in females.

Investigations should include thyroxine, TSH and thyroid antibodies. Elevated TSH demonstrates primary hypothyroidism. If thyroxine levels are normal in the presence of raised TSH, then it is described as compensated hypothyroidism, but may progress to overt hypothyroidism (low thyroxine levels). Antibodies to thyroglobulin and thyroid peroxidase (TPO) are detectable in 95% of cases. TPO antibodies are more sensitive and specific. Bone age is delayed. This patient had a TSH of >150 mU/l (normal <6 mU/l) and a thyroxine level below 20 nmol/l (normal 70-140 nmol/l).

Treatment should be commenced with L-Thyroxine at a dose of 100 mcg/m². Dosage will need to be adjusted according to symptoms and biochemical testing. Follow-up to monitor growth and puberty is essential.

CASE 10.2

A 7-year-old Somali boy was referred to the paediatric surgical team for drainage of a large abscess on his left buttock. A history was difficult to obtain as the family had recently come to the UK from Somalia, but, with the help of an interpreter, it transpired that the boy was prone to recurrent abscesses in various sites of his body. On three previous occasions, he had had to be admitted to hospital for surgical drainage of the abscess. Following the abscess's successful drainage, the child was treated with a 5-day course of i.v. flucloxacillin (as pus from the abscess revealed a growth of *Staphylococcus aureus*), and the boy was discharged home, to be reviewed by the paediatric medical team in the out-patient clinic in 4 weeks' time.

What diagnosis is the history suggestive of?

SELECT *TWO* ANSWERS ONLY

i. Defect in cellular immunity
ii. T-cell deficiency
iii. SCID
iv. Agammaglobulinaemia
v. Neutrophil disorder
vi. IgA deficiency
vii. Phagocytic disorder

v. Neutrophil disorder

vii. Phagocytic disorder

In suspected immune deficiency, a full history is important, especially of gingivitis, mouth ulcers and fever, and any family history of recurrent serious infections suggestive of immune disorder. Examination should include height and weight, and evidence of failure to thrive. Knowing when and how to investigate is important. Until 5 years of age, normal children have up to 12 respiratory infections per year. Frequency is influenced by: presence of older siblings, child-care attendance and exposure to tobacco smoke. The child is likely normal but prone to infections if: infections are mild, acute and probably viral; recovery is usually without sequelae; growth pattern is normal; infections are restricted to a single site suggest local obstruction, i.e. an anatomical problem. This history is highly suggestive of a neutrophil problem. Investigations should be in two stages. A large number of immune function tests are available. It is therefore, important to choose the most appropriate. After a detailed history and a careful clinical examination, an idea should be gained of which immunity is involved:

1. Cellular immunity:
   a. Cells involved: T-lymphocytes and CD4 and CD8 cells; T-cell help is required for B-cells to function normally
   b. Clinical picture: pneumocystis carinii pneumonia, persistent oral candidiasis, persistent diarrhoea (rotavirus or other viruses), failure to thrive, for example severe combined immunodeficiency disease or HIV

2. Humoral immunity:
   a. Cells involved: B-cells from the bone marrow; these produce antibodies but need help from T-cells
   b. Clinical picture: sino-pulmonary infections (otitis media, sinusitis, etc.), especially with encapsulated bacteria, and serious infections such as osteomyelitis, septic arthritis and meningitis

3. Complement system:
   a. A series of proteins that interact sequentially on the cell surface in a cascade, starting with either the classical or alternative pathway and leading to a common pathway that generates chemotactic factors and opsonins, and causes cell lysis
   b. Clinical picture: recurrent bacteraemia and meningitis (especially neisserial infections)

4. Phagocytic system:
   a. Cells involved: neutrophils
   b. Clinical picture: boils, furunculosis, mouth ulcers, gingivitis and deep-seated abscesses. There is increased susceptibility to Staph aureus, Gram-negative bacilli, such as Pseudomonas and fungi, for example Aspergillus

5. Natural killer cell function:
   a. Cells involved: natural killer cells kill virus-infected cells, some microorganisms and tumour cells spontaneously, being stimulated by interferon
   b. Clinical picture: this is important in recovery from herpes infection (HSV, CMV and herpes zoster virus), especially when haemophagocytosis is suspected

Table 10.2.

Investigations	How performed	Interpretation
First line		
Neutrophil count	Blood film	Congenital and acquired neutropaenia
Serum IgE	Nephelometry or ELISA	Very high in hyper-IgE syndrome
Second line		
NBT (nitroblue tetrazolium test)	Specialised laboratory	Chronic granulomatous disease
Neutrophil function tests, e.g. chemotaxis, chemoluminescence	Specialised laboratory	If NBT is −ve and neutrophil defect is suspected
Weekly neutrophil count for 6/52	Blood film	Suspected cyclical neutropaenia (fever ± infection ± mouth ulcers every 3 weeks)
CD11, CD18	Fluorescent-activated cell sorter (FACS)	Suspected leukocyte adhesion defect (delayed separation of umbilical cord, severe early infection)

CASE 10.3

A 10-year-old is brought to A&E by his grandparents with complaints of sudden high fever, lethargy and drowsiness. While being assessed, he has a prolonged generalised seizure. He remains unconscious despite cessation of the seizure with diazepam. He is admitted with a diagnosis of probable meningoencephalitis. Nursing staff discover that he attends a boarding school. His parents work along the East African coast as missionaries and he has recently spent the Christmas holidays with them.

What further investigations are essential for this child as a guide for immediate action?

SELECT *THREE* ANSWERS ONLY
   i. CXR
  ii. Thick and thin blood films
 iii. FBC
  iv. Ammonia
   v. Blood glucose
  vi. Calcium
 vii. Stool for ova, cysts and parasites
viii. Stool for M,C& S

ANSWERS TO CASE 10.3

ii. Thick and thin blood films
iii. FBC
v. Blood glucose

Foremost, hypoglycaemia must be looked for and treated appropriately. Other initial laboratory tests should include FBC, U&E, blood gas analysis, a blood culture and repeated blood films for malaria parasites. A lumbar puncture should only be performed if there are no clinical indicators of raised intracranial pressure.

The blood film in this case was reported as "scanty falciparum malaria parasites seen". This suggests a diagnosis of cerebral malaria. Although a heavy parasitaemia is associated with an increased risk of severe anaemia, a scanty parasitaemia may follow tissue seques-tration of mature parasites or partial treatment. Parasites in the blood film, however, do not rule out meningitis or encephalitis. A lumbar puncture for CSF analysis is always mandatory.

The convulsion and subsequent coma could be due to hypoglycaemia, deranged meta-bolic status, particularly severe acidosis or the disease process itself. Hypoglycaemia is a poor prognostic marker in severe malaria.

The definitive treatment is an antimalarial drug. The correct drug, dosage and route are important. The decision of which drug to use is best guided by national policy which considers known local drug sensitivities. Quinine (i.v.) remains the drug of choice for the treatment of cerebral malaria, although novel drugs are available includ-ing the artemesinin derivatives. In addition, broad-spectrum antibiotics for possible meningitis and septicaemia must be commenced until definitive diagnosis is made. Control of intractable seizures may be difficult. Phenytoin is often effective. Anti-pyretics are used for control of fever.

Supportive treatment is of paramount importance. Blood glucose, parasite clearance, haemoglobin, renal function, and conscious level must be monitored.

Transfusion is only indicated if symptomatic, otherwise the anaemia will often correct spontaneously. Thrombocytopaenia is common in falciparum infection but is not linked to a poor prognosis and recovers spontaneously, so that, unless there is a bleeding dia-thesis, platelet transfusion is rarely necessary.

At follow-up, these patients require careful examination for neurological sequelae, including hemiparesis, blindness, cerebellar defects and seizures.

CASE 10.4

1. Asthma
2. Bronchiectasis
3. TB
4. CF
5. Pneumocystis carinii
6. VSD
7. Gastroesophageal reflux
8. ASD
9. Bronchiolitis obliterans
10. Mitral stenosis

For each of the following case scenarios select the most likely diagnosis from the list above:

a. A 3-year-old boy presents with worsening cough and breathlessness of 3 weeks' duration. He has always been prone to infections. When he was 2 years old he had chicken pox for 4 weeks. On examination, he has an emaciated appearance, his weight is below the 0.4th centile, he has a temperature of 37.6°C and he has generalised crepitations on auscultation of his chest. A blood count shows severe lymphopenia. *PCP*

b. A 14 years old Malaysian boy living in a small village presented at a local clinic with a history of increased breathlessness over the past few weeks. He has a history of previous illness and was admitted to hospital for 2 weeks when he was 8 years old. On examination the apex beat is located in the 5th left intercostal space, mid-clavicular line and there is an audible murmur. *mitral stenosis*

c. A 6-week-old girl had an uncomplicated birth at term following a normal pregnancy. At 6 weeks' of age she was admitted with a cough, fever, increased breathlessness and an increased oxygen requirement. She vomited, became breathless and deteriorated 48 h after admission. On examination she was not dysmorphic. Heart sounds were normal. Her respiratory rate was 60 bpm and she was recessing. There was biphasic wheeze heard throughout her lung fields. Her oxygen saturations were 90% in air. A CXR showed consolidation of the right middle lobe. She was commenced on low flow oxygen, intravenous fluids and broad-spectrum antibiotics after appropriate cultures were taken. She responded well and feeds were recommenced after 48 h. After a further 48 hours she relapsed and required intubation and ventilation again. *GORD*

a. 5. Pneumocystis carinii

Pneumocystis carinii causes a diffuse pneumonitis with fever, tachypnoea, hypoxaemia and bilateral diffuse infiltrates on X-ray. It often leads to respiratory failure and the need for intubation and ventilation. Pneumocystis carinii pneumonia (PCP) occurs almost exclusively in the immunocompromised host. Children with congenital or acquired immune deficiency syndrome (AIDS), and recipients of suppressive therapy in the treatment of malignancies or after organ transplantation are at high risk.

PCP is an AIDS-defining illness. It is the most common opportunistic life-threatening lung infection in infants with perinatally acquired HIV disease. PCP in the HIV patient can occur at any time, but usually presents during the first year of life. More that 70% of healthy individuals have antibodies by the age of 4 years.

b. 10. Mitral stenosis

Symptoms of mitral stenosis may appear within 3-4 years of rheumatic fever or may be delayed for decades. Symptoms depend on the presence of pulmonary hypertension with low cardiac output (weakness, fatigue), and then, when the right ventricle fails, symptoms of congestive cardiac failure (hepatomegaly, peripheral oedema).

c. 7. Gastroesophageal reflux

This history is consistent with aspiration secondary to a diagnosis of gastroesophageal reflux. Other causes of aspiration which must be considered include tracheo-oesophageal fistula, oropharyngeal incoordination or laryngeal cleft. Investigations may include passage of the nasogastric tube, a pH probe study, a barium swallow, videofluoroscopy and feeding assessment, bronchoscopy, laryngoscopy and endoscopy.

Gastroesophageal reflux may be treated medically but sometimes if severe, may require fundoplication and gastrostomy feeding.

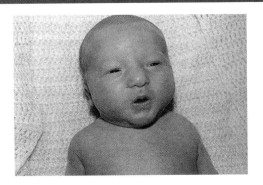

Fig 10.5

A 3-day-old baby boy was reviewed on the post-natal ward following an episode of generalised "jerking". He had been born at term in good condition by spontaneous vertex delivery (SVD) and there were no clinical concerns prior to this episode. On examination, he was noted to be dysmorphic (Fig. 10.5) and jittery.

Serum biochemistry was as follows:
  Na 135 mmol/l
  Ca 1.27 mmol/l
  PO$_4$ 3.35 mmol/l
  Mg 0.8 mmol/l
  Glucose 3.6 mmol/l

a. What is the likely diagnosis?
   SELECT *ONE* ANSWER ONLY
   i. Beckwith–Wiedemann syndrome
   ii. Russell–Silver syndrome
   iii. Autosomal dominant neonatal seizures
   iv. DiGeorge syndrome
   v. William's syndrome

b. What other investigations should be requested?
   SELECT *TWO* ANSWERS ONLY
   i. EEG
   ii. Organic acids
   iii. Echocardiogram
   iv. Parathyroid hormone
   v. Ammonia
   vi. Lumbar puncture

ANSWERS TO CASE 10.5

a. iv. DiGeorge syndrome
b. iii. Echocardiogram
   iv. Parathyroid hormone

These results demonstrate low calcium with high phosphate. The likely diagnosis is hypocalcaemic hypoparathyroidism as part of DiGeorge syndrome.

This can be confirmed by fluorescent in-situ hybridization (FISH) analysis for chromosomal deletion at 22q11.2.

Further investigations should include an echocardiogram for evidence of congenital heart disease, a CXR/chest ultrasound scan for absence of the thymus, T-lymphocyte subsets and PTH levels.

The DiGeorge syndrome forms part of the constellation of abnormalities collectively termed CATCH 22 (cardiac defects, abnormal facies, thymic hypoplasia, cleft palate, hypocalcaemia). These occur as a result of maldevelopment of the third and fourth pharyngeal pouches in early embryonic life.

A spectrum of clinical findings occurs. This classically includes conotruncal cardiac abnormalities, abnormal facial appearance (downward slanting palpebral fissures, a small chin, broad forehead and abnormal ears), absence of the thymus (with resultant T-cell-mediated immune deficiency), and absence or hypoplasia of the parathyroid glands (leading to hypocalcaemia).

Less well recognised are learning, speech, feeding and psychiatric disorders. The 22q11.2. deletion can be inherited as an autosomal dominant disorder (as in this family) or arise as a de-novo deletion or translocation.

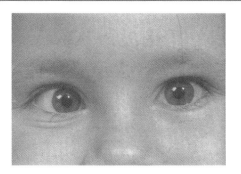

Fig 10.6

A 3-year-old boy presented with a 4-day history of being generally unwell: lethargic with a decreased oral intake. On day 2 of the illness he developed a sticky right eye. His GP prescribed chloromycetin eye drops for conjunctivitis. Hours after using the drops his mother noticed a squint; she assumed this was due to the treatment, which she continued. She also noticed that he was very unsteady on his feet. He was no better 3 days later and the GP referred the child to A&E. On arrival the boy had a GCS of 14, was irritable, lying curled up on his side with his neck hyperextended, and was afebrile, pulse 119, blood pressure 95/55 with a right-sided 6th cranial nerve palsy. The child was uncooperative for the remaining neurological assessment; however, reflexes seemed normal but with equivocal plantar responses. The fundi could not be visualised. FBC, U&Es, blood cultures and serum for virology were taken.

a. What are the possible diagnoses?
   SELECT *TWO* ANSWERS ONLY
   i. Orbital cellulitis
   ii. Subdural haemorrhage
   iii. Intracranial space-occupying lesion
   iv. Meningitis
   v. Benign intracranial hypertension

b. What further tests would you want initially?
   SELECT *TWO* ANSWERS ONLY
   i. Lumbar puncture
   ii. Ophthalmological review
   iii. Urine toxicology
   iv. CT scan
   v. EEG
   vi. Serum calcium and magnesium

c. What treatment would you initiate?
   SELECT *TWO* ANSWERS ONLY
   i. Steroids
   ii. i.v. benzylpenicillin
   iii. i.v. acyclovir
   iv. Mannitol
   v. i.v. cefotaxime

ANSWERS TO CASE 10.6

a. iii. Intracranial space-occupying lesion
   iv. Meningitis
b. i. Lumbar puncture
   iv. CT scan
c. iii. i.v. acyclovir
    v. i.v. cefotaxime

This previously well 3-year-old child presented with a vague history of being generally unwell with ataxia and a new squint. The positive findings on examination were extreme irritability, the neck hyperextension and the squint. There was no history of fever and vital signs were stable.

After the initial bloods were taken he began on i.v. cefotaxime and acyclovir to cover bacterial meningitis and herpes encephalitis. However, his signs fitted well with a space-occupying lesion and he underwent urgent CT scan under general anaesthetic. This was normal with no evidence of raised intracranial pressure. Whilst under anaesthetic, his fundi were visualised (normal) and a lumbar puncture was performed. The CSF contained 840 white cells (80% neutrophils) and 60 red cells. CSF glucose was 2.4 mmol/l (serum 5.5 mmol/l) and protein was 40 g/l. Multiple other investigations were done to look for an acute cause of his ataxia including a metabolic screen, thyroid function and Lyme disease serology.

After 24 h he was markedly better. Apart from the squint he was back to normal by day 4. Intravenous antibiotics and anti-virals were stopped after 1 week. At this time the CSF PCR result was received which was positive for meningococcus.

Unilateral cranial nerve palsy is a recognised complication of bacterial meningitis but most commonly the facial nerve is involved. The palsies tend to be transient.

CASE 10.7

A boy of 7 years attends a clinic showing rigidity in his routines and getting upset when they are changed. He gets agitated if he misses programmes on television and gets temper tantrums when he is asked to do things or to change his routine. He insists that stories have to be read to him in a particular way. On enquiry it is clear that he was late in showing imaginative play; however, his early development was otherwise normal. He lacks close friends and when attempting to play with his peer-group, he insists on doing things in a certain way. If rules are changed he is unhappy and sometimes aggressive. He avoids eye contact, his language tends to be formal and pedantic and he does not follow conversations well. His speech is loud, fast and often delivered in a monotone way reflecting his interests at length without regard to the listener's attention. He has acquired extensive knowledge about aeroplanes and other circumscribed interests while his application to school work is inconsistent, despite above average ability on formal assessments.

What diagnosis is suggested from this information?

SELECT THE *MOST APPROPRIATE* ANSWER

   i. Dyspraxia
   ii. Obsessive-compulsive disorder
   iii. Autism
   iv. Asperger syndrome
   v. Rett's syndrome
   vi. Childhood-onset schizophrenia

ANSWER TO CASE 10.7

iv. Asperger syndrome (AS)

The following are the criteria for the diagnosis of AS (DSM-IV):

1. Severe and sustained impairment in social interaction manifested by at least two of the following: impairment of non-verbal behaviour, for example eye-to-eye gaze, facial expression, body postures and gestures to regulate social interaction; failure to develop peer relationships; lack of spontaneous seeking to share enjoyment, interests, or achievement with other individuals; and lack of social or emotional reciprocity
2. Restricted repetitive and stereotyped pattern of behaviour, interests, and activities as manifested by at least one of the following: encompassing preoccupation with at least one stereotyped and restricted pattern of interest that is abnormal either in intensity or focus; inflexible adherence to specific, non-functional routines or rituals; stereotyped and repetitive motor mannerisms; and persistent preoccupation with parts of objects
3. Clinically significant impairment in social, occupational or other areas of functioning
4. No significant delays in cognitive development, in the development of self-help skills, adaptive behaviour (other than social interaction) and curiosity about the environment
5. No clinically significant delay in language development
6. Criteria not met for other specific pervasive disorders or schizophrenia

Other conditions to be considered include other pervasive developmental disorders such as childhood disintegrative disorder, autism or pervasive disorders not otherwise specified. In a girl, Rett syndrome might be a differential diagnosis. All pervasive developmental disorders are characterised by impairment of reciprocal social interaction, verbal and non-verbal communication skills or the presence of stereotyped behaviour, interests and activities. Further differential diagnoses include schizoid personality disorder, obsessive-compulsive disorder and very rarely, childhood-onset schizophrenia.

AS is a specific condition on the autism "spectrum" and is more common in males. In contrast to childhood autism, there are no significant delays in early language development. Symptoms in autistic disorders have to be present prior to the age of 3 years; AS is generally diagnosed later, typically in mid-childhood. Childhood disintegrative disorder is defined by developmental regression after at least 2 years of normal development. AS and OCD share repetitive and stereotyped patterns of interests in their diagnostic criterion. Individuals with AS exhibit qualitative impairment in social interaction and a more restricted pattern of interests. AS is distinguished from schizoid personality disorder by stereotyped behaviours and interests and by a more severely impaired social interaction.

CASE 10.8

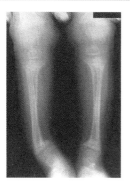

Fig 10.8.A

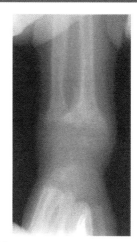

Fig 10.8.B

A 2-year-old is referred for a medical examination by his GP and social services, after a deformity of his right ankle was noted. The parents had no explanation to offer. He is still breast fed and there have been concerns raised previously about his mildly delayed motor development. He is one of three children who live with their parents and other families in a large isolated house. The health visitor, who is not allowed to visit, describes their lifestyle as "alternative".

On examination he is well grown, with no signs of trauma. He has swollen wrists and an obvious abnormality of his right ankle. X-rays are taken (see Figs 10.8.A & 10.8.B).

a. What features are shown on the X-rays?
   SELECT *TWO* ANSWERS ONLY
   i. Poor bone mineralisation
   ii. Pathological fracture
   iii. Rachitic rosary
   iv. Delayed bone age
   v. Metaphyseal splaying
   vi. Callous formation

b. What investigations would you do to help confirm the diagnosis?
   SELECT *TWO* ANSWERS ONLY
   i. Bone scan
   ii. Serum phosphate
   iii. Urinary phosphate
   iv. Skeletal survey
   v. DEXA scan
   vi. Serum uric acid

c. What is the major danger of treatment?
   SELECT *ONE* ANSWER ONLY
   i. Secondary hypoparathyroidism
   ii. Seizures
   iii. Nephrocalcinosis
   iv. Hypocalcaemia
   v. Tetany

ANSWERS TO CASE 10.8

a. i. Poor bone mineralisation
    v. Metaphyseal splaying
b. ii. Serum phosphate
    v. DEXA scan
c. iii. Nephrocalcinosis

The X-rays show the main features of rickets:
Generalised poor bone mineralization
Deformity of long bones and delayed development of epiphyses
"Cupping", "fraying" and "splaying" of the metaphysis (i.e. concave, irregular metaphyseal margins with a greater than normal diameter)

The diagnosis of "rickets" is confirmed by finding a high serum alkaline phosphatase, a low phosphate and low/normal calcium. Rickets is further classified in Table 10.8.1.

In the case described, results were consistent with vitamin D deficient rickets. Further history confirmed risk factors for vitamin D deficiency:
Prolonged breast feeding
Minimal exposure to sunlight
Poor dietary sources of vitamin D

It is important to exclude malabsorption, and screen other family members.

Treatment consists of high dose vitamin D (1000–5000 iu/day) until alkaline phosphatase is in normal range, then vitamin D intake maintained at "normal" level of 400 iu/day. Success of treatment is confirmed by biochemical parameters returning to normal. A repeat X-ray will show radiographic evidence of improvement.

The risk of high dose vitamin D is hypercalcaemia and consequent nephrocalcinosis – it is important to monitor serum calcium levels during treatment.

Table 10.8.1

	25-HCC	1,25- DHCC	PO$_4$	PTH
Vitamin D deficiency (i.e. lack of dietary vit. D, lack of sunlight, malabsorption)	Low	Low	Low	High/normal
Vitamin D dependent rickets Type I (i.e. defect in Vit D metabolism)	Normal	Low	Low	Increased/normal
Vitamin D dependent rickets Type II (i.e. vit D receptors "defective")	Normal	Normal	Low	Increased/normal
Vitamin D resistant (hypophosphataemic) rickets (i.e. X-linked hypophosphataemic rickets, renal PO$_4$ loss – Fanconi's, etc.)	Normal	Normal	Very low	Normal

CASE 10.9

A 3-year-old girl was admitted with a short history of pyrexia, vomiting and a possible seizure at home. Her mother gave a history of previous illnesses associated with drowsiness and vomiting. She had mild developmental delay and poor speech. On examination, she was unrousable. A full infection screen including lumbar puncture was negative.

Initial bloods showed:

Hb 12.7 g/dl	Na 138 mmol/l
WCC 17 × 10⁹/l	K 3.8 mmol/l
Platelets 270 × 10⁹/l	Urea 1.4 mmol/l
CRP 77	Creatinine 62 μmol/l
Glucose 4.5 mmol/l	LFTs normal
Ammonia 412 μmol/l	Lactate 3.98 mmol/l

Venous gas: pH 7.411, pCO_2 34.6 mmHg, bicarbonate 22.9 mmol/l
Cranial CT was normal

a. What is the likely diagnosis?
SELECT *ONE* ANSWER ONLY
  i. Urea cycle disorder
  ii. Mitochondrial disorder
  iii. Reye's syndrome
  iv. Organic aciduria
  v. Medium chain acyl-CoA dehydrogenase deficiency

b. What treatment may be needed?
SELECT *THREE* ANSWERS ONLY
  i. Forced alkaline diuresis
  ii. Stop protein intake acutely
  iii. Restrict protein intake to 2 g/kg/day
  iv. Dialysis or haemofiltration
  v. Sodium benzoate
  vi. Calcium benzoate
  vii. Dexamethasone

ANSWERS TO CASE 10.9

a.   i. Urea cycle disorder
b.   ii. Stop protein intake acutely
    iv. Dialysis or haemofiltration
    v. Sodium benzoate

The diagnosis is a urea cycle disorder, which is suggested by the high ammonia (normal level 10-47 µmol/l), the metabolic alkalosis, and the low urea.

The differential diagnosis of hyperammonaemia would include an organic aciduria and Reye syndrome.

The history given of recurrent illnesses associated with vomiting and drowsiness should prompt a search for underlying inborn errors of metabolism. In infants, feeding problems, vomiting, failure to thrive and chronic neurological symptoms may be noted. Episodes of encephalopathy occur with vomiting, drowsiness, ataxia and irritability, progressing to coma. Seizures and developmental delay are common. Because of the importance of identifying treatable metabolic disorders, early investigation of patients presenting stuporose or obtunded should not be delayed.

Management involves resuscitation: ABC. Protein intake should be stopped immediately. Fits should be appropriately treated. Treatment of hyperammonaemia may involve dialysis or haemofiltration, especially if the ammonia is over 400 µmol/l. Sodium benzoate, sodium phenylacetate and arginine are also used.

Other investigations include plasma and urine amino acids, which may show characteristic changes. Liver biopsy allows precise identification of the enzyme deficiency in the urea cycle disorders. This girl had carbamyl phosphate synthetase deficiency.

CASE 10.10

A 2-year-old boy, with recurrent glue ear, who was fully immunised, including *Haemophilus influenzae* type b (Hib vaccine), was admitted with a right-sided preseptal cellulitis. His corneal swab grew *Haemophilus influenzae* type b.

How should this child's immunological status be further assessed?

SELECT *ONE* ANSWER ONLY

   i. Hib antibodies checked, and reimmunised if low
  ii. Serum immunoglobulins, and investigate further if low
 iii. No antibody check necessary, but revaccinate
 iv. No investigations and no vaccination necessary

ANSWER TO CASE 10.10

iv. No investigations and no vaccination necessary

No assessment necessary. Hib vaccine protects against capsulated strain infections only, such as seen in meningitis, osteomyelitis, and epiglottitis. It does not protect against otitis media and conjunctivitis, which are caused by uncapsulated strains. This is because the vaccine is made by conjugating polysaccharide capsular antigen to a carrier protein. This improves vaccine immunogenicity, especially in children less than a year. Similar conjugation techniques were used to produce the meningococcal C vaccine.

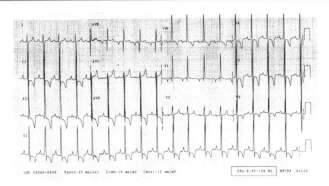

Fig 10.11

An 8-year-old girl presented with a 6-month history of increasing lethargy and weight loss of 4 kg. Her parents had noted that she had cool extremities and blue cheeks and lips. Recently, she had been fainting at school following exercise and she was also noted to have facial tics and abnormal arm movements. She had been adopted at the age of 6 months and little was known about her perinatal and postnatal period. She had been under follow-up for global developmental delay and learning difficulties. Her only admission to the hospital was at the age of 9 months with bronchiolitis. On examination, she was not dysmorphic. Both her weight and height were below the 0.4th centile. Her lips appeared to be mildly dusky but she was not clubbed. A right parasternal heave was palpable. On auscultation, her first heart sound was normal and her second was accentuated but no murmurs were heard. Her chest was clear and only the liver tip was palpable. Her ECG is shown.

What does the ECG show?

SELECT *THREE* ANSWERS ONLY
   i. Left ventricular hypertrophy
  ii. Right axis deviation
 iii. Right ventricular hypertrophy
  iv. Superior axis
   v. ST elevation
  vi. Left axis deviation
 vii. Right atrial enlargement
viii. Long QT interval

ii. Right axis deviation
iii. Right ventricular hypertrophy
vii. Right atrial enlargement

ECG shows right axis deviation, right atrial enlargement and right ventricular hypertrophy; very unusual in a child of her age indicating elevated right-sided pressures. Investigations helpful in primary pulmonary hypertension (PPH) diagnosis: CXR, echo, V/Q scan, thrombophilia screen, autoantibodies, ESR, FBC+film, and chromosomes.

PPH may be primary or secondary to underlying disease:
1. Cardiac causes: supramitral ring/web, untreated AVSD
2. Respiratory causes: chronic lung disease, CF, chronic upper airway obstruction (large tonsils and adenoids)
3. Thromboembolic cause: iatrogenic, coagulopathy, schistosomiasis
4. Connective tissue disorder: systemic lupus erythematosus

PPH is raised mean pulmonary arterial pressure >25 mmHg at rest (>30 mmHg during exercise) with no identifiable cause; rapidly progressive, it causes disabling symptoms, leading to death if untreated. Non-specific symptoms are usual: breathlessness (most common), chest pain and syncope. Often 3 years pass between first symptoms and diagnosis. CXR, ECG and respiratory referral should be requested; the former is usually abnormal (85%), showing enlarged proximal pulmonary arteries ("proximal pruning") and the ECG shows right ventricular hypertrophy. Supportive treatment rather than curative is usual:

- Oxygen therapy: hypoxaemia causes pulmonary vasoconstriction and thus worsening of pulmonary hypertension
- Anticoagulation: reduces pulmonary arterial thrombosis and hypercoagulable state present in pulmonary hypertension
- Vasodilator therapy: using Ca antagonists, which cause pulmonary and systemic vasodilatation
- Long-term prostacyclin therapy: potent endogenous vasodilator, which inhibits platelet aggregation, thought to be associated with remodelling pulmonary vascular bed, with subsequent reduction in endothelial cell injury and hypercoagulability
- Atrial septostomy: a palliative procedure, which acts as a "blow off valve" during hypertensive crises, the child shunts right to left across the atrial communication becoming cyanotic, but maintaining cardiac output.
- Lung transplantation improves quality of life and survival.

A P wave of >2.5 mm tall reflects right atrial enlargement. A P wave of >120 ms in duration reflects left atrial enlargement.

Right ventricular hypertrophy is demonstrated by:
- right axis deviation
- neonatal R/S progression across the chest leads after the newborn period (i.e. dominant R in V1 and dominant S in V6)
- abnormally large R wave in V1 or S in V6
- Upright T wave in V1 after day 3 and under 6 years of age

A 14-year-old Asian girl was referred by her GP to the paediatric surgical team with a diagnosis of possible acute appendicitis. She had been experiencing recurrent bouts of colicky abdominal pain (mainly right sided), loose stools and loss of appetite for the preceding 2 days. Examination revealed a pale, thin girl who was obviously unwell and in pain. She was mildly febrile and normotensive, with a pulse rate of 90 bpm. Her abdomen was generally tender on palpation, more so in the right iliac fossa, but there was no guarding or rebound tenderness. She had numerous mouth ulcers. On plotting the girl's height and weight, she was below the third centile for both. On further questioning, her father mentioned that she had been experiencing these recurrent bouts of abdominal pain and diarrhoea for the previous 6 months.

What is the most probable diagnosis for this girl?

SELECT *ONE* ANSWER ONLY

  i. Irritable bowel syndrome
 ii. Sub acute appendicitis
iii. Vitamin B deficiency
 iv. Ulcerative colitis
  v. Lymphoma
 vi. Crohn's disease

Questions and Answers for the New Format Exam

vi. Crohn's disease

Any history of weight loss, rectal bleeding, urgency, tenesmus, peri-anal symptoms and nausea and vomiting, as well as joint pains, skin rashes and episodes of unexplained fever should be established. It is also important to enquire about whether the girl has started to develop signs of puberty, i.e. whether she has started the menarche.

The most probable diagnosis for this girl is Crohn's disease. Investigations should include:

1. Blood tests: FBC, acute phase reactants (CRP, ferritin), ESR, serum and red cell folate, serum vitamin B12, LFTs and serum albumin, serology for Yersinia enteropathica and Entamoeba histolytica
2. Stool tests: stool microscopy of fresh stool (ova, cysts, parasites, Giardia and amoebae), stool culture (Salmonella, Shigella, Campylobacter, enteropathogenic E. coli and Clostridium difficile toxin)
3. Imaging: abdominal ultrasound, barium meal and follow-through, white cell scan
4. Upper gastrointestinal endoscopy and colonoscopy (with ileoscopy)

Crohn's disease presents usually over the age of 10 years, but more children are presenting earlier. In childhood and adolescence the disease often manifests similarly to adults, but children sometimes present without GI symptoms, showing only growth failure, pyrexia of unknown origin and pseudo-appendicitis. Diagnosis is often delayed by up to 2 years, especially with primary systemic features such as growth failure, thought to be caused by malnutrition as well as the inflammatory process. Inflammation leads to the release of tumour necrosis factor-alpha, postulated to have a direct effect on the epiphyseal growth plates. GI symptoms include: abdominal pain, anorexia, nausea, vomiting and diarrhoea. Abdominal pain (often brought on by eating) is characteristically peri-umbilical and colicky. Anorexia may be so severe that anorexia nervosa is sometimes diagnosed. Chronic constipation can also be an important feature. Vomiting and diarrhoea may have an acute onset and suggest acute gastroenteritis. Differentiation from ulcerative colitis may be difficult if bloody diarrhoea results from colonic involvement. Physical examination may reveal retarded growth and development, delayed puberty, facial pallor with characteristically dark skin beneath the eyes, frank oral ulceration and angular cheilitis. Other feature include a palpable abdominal mass, painless anal fissures and a peri-anal abscess or a fistula-in-ano. Children may present with a severe attack and a "toxic" appearance with pallor, tachycardia and swinging fever. A secure diagnosis depends on histological findings (total colonoscopy, with entry into the ileum, usually revealing sarcoid-like, non-caseating granulomata in the mucosa or submucosa); barium meal and follow-through should be performed to visualise the ileum adequately. Upper GI endoscopy may be used to differentiate between Crohn's disease and ulcerative colitis.

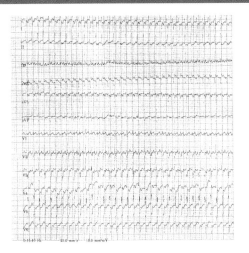

Fig 10.13

A 10-week-old boy presented with a 3-day history of being off his feeds and 2 days of vomiting. He had had several self-limiting episodes of pallor and tachypnoea over the previous few days. He had been born at full term and was being breast fed and making appropriate developmental progress. On examination, he was pale and sweaty with a delayed capillary refill time. His heart rate was over 240 bpm. An ECG was obtained.

a. What does the ECG show?
   SELECT *TWO* ANSWERS ONLY
   i. Superior axis
   ii. Ventricular tachycardia
   iii. 1 : 1 AV conduction
   iv. Sinus tachycardia
   v. Supraventricular tachycardia
   vi. Broad complex tachycardia

b. What condition, diagnosable on ECG, are these findings associated with?
   SELECT *ONE* ANSWER ONLY
   i. Wolff–Parkinson–White (WPW) syndrome
   ii. Atrioventricular septal defect
   iii. Salbutamol toxicity
   iv. Hypertrophic obstructive cardiomyopathy
   v. Pericarditis

ANSWERS TO CASE 10.13

a. iii. 1 : 1 AV conduction
   v. Supraventricular tachycardia
b. i. Wolff–Parkinson–White (WPW) syndrome

The differential diagnosis from the history alone must include sepsis and cardiac failure, as well as a cardiac arrhythmia. The ECG here shows supraventricular tachycardia with a rate of 300 bpm, a narrow QRS complex with 1 : 1 AV conduction.

SVT is the most common abnormal arrhythmia in infancy and childhood, and the majority of children have structurally normal hearts. In infants, most attacks occur before 6 months of age and the prognosis is excellent. Attacks may be transient and undetected, and if attacks last for more than 24 h, heart failure usually ensues and treatment becomes urgent. In older children, episodes may recur over many years and may be refractory to treatment necessitating ablation of the accessory connection.

Treatment is dependent on the presence of shock on presentation. If shock is present then cardioversion is the treatment of choice. Cardioversion in an unconscious or anaesthetised child is given using a synchronised shock delivered at 0.5/1/2 J/kg. Other treatments include vagal manoeuvres, i.v. adenosine, i.v. digoxin and flecainide. Vagal manoeuvres, such as eliciting the diving reflex by submerging the face into icy water, can be very effective in aborting an attack. Adenosine given in an i.v. bolus acts to prevent conduction through the AV node. Intravenous digoxin or flecainide can be used under the supervision of a cardiologist.

SVT is associated with WPW syndrome. A large proportion of infants and children with paroxysmal SVT show ECG features of WPW syndrome – a short PR interval, broad QRS complex and delta wave. The accessory pathway bypasses junctional tissue that allows a circuit to be formed that facilitates re-entry tachycardia.

The accessory pathway may go from the left atrium to the left ventricle (type A) simulating right bundle branch block or from the right atrium to the right ventricle (type B) simulating a left bundle branch block pattern.

CASE 10.14

A 5-month-old Caucasian baby girl was admitted to the local hospital with a 2-week history of being generally unwell with intermittent pyrexia. On the day of referral to the hospital she had a generalised tonic clonic convulsion. She was born at term by normal vaginal delivery. The mother had been in contact with her partner, who had a chronic cough. Initial investigations done showed:

Hb 11.6 g/dl
WBC 27.5 × 10⁹/l
Neutrophils 12.9 × 10⁹/l
Lymphocytes 11.6 × 10⁹/l
Platelets 595 × 10⁹/l
CRP 22.5 mg/l (<10)
Blood glucose 4 mmol/l
CSF gross – slightly turbid
CSF Microscopy 115 WBC/mm³ (80% polymorphs and 20% lymphocytes)
CSF Protein 1.7 g/l
CSF Glucose 0.2 mmol/l
CT scan – bilateral dilated ventricles

What diagnosis should be considered most likely?

SELECT *ONE* ANSWER ONLY
  i. CNS vasculitis
 ii. Medulloblastoma
iii. Cerebral leukaemic infiltration
 iv. Herpes simplex encephalitis
  v. Viral meningitis
 vi. Tuberculous meningitis

ANSWER TO CASE 10.14

vi. Tuberculous meningitis

Bacterial or tuberculous meningitis (TBM) would be your main differential diagnosis with the CSF findings and history of contact with partner having a chronic cough. The CSF findings show low glucose, mildly elevated protein and mixed cells with polymorphonuclear cells predominating at this stage.

Further tests to assist in making the diagnosis include CSF Gram-stain and Ziehl–Nielson stain to look for acid-fast bacilli (AFB), CSF culture for bacteria and mycobacterium tuberculosis, Mantoux test, PCR for mycobacterial DNA, CXR and early-morning nasogastric aspirates. Mantoux test is positive in up to 90% of TBM and therefore is very useful. Mycobacterial DNA in CSF may be a more sensitive test than CSF stain and culture as AFB are seen in only 25% of CSF smears and about 50% of CSF will grow the bacilli after several weeks. Sensitivity for DNA PCR is about 90%.

Until the diagnosis is confirmed the child should be commenced on broad-spectrum antibiotics and antituberculous drugs. Four-drug antitubercular treatment with steroids should be commenced. Postinfective hydrocephalus may need shunting. Public health notification and screening of family are important additional measures.

This patient had tuberculous meningitis. The prognosis is related to the patient's condition at the time of treatment. In the early stages of the disease (i.e. prodromal phase) a 100% cure and a low incidence of sequelae can be anticipated. In cases where neurological signs and symptoms are present prior to commencement of treatment approximately 50% survivors show neurological defects. In those presenting with altered consciousness levels a 50% survival has been reported despite treatment and most survivors have permanent handicap.

Tuberculosis constitutes a major cause of death worldwide. An estimated 1.3 million cases of tuberculosis and 450 000 associated deaths occur annually in children. Recent times have seen a resurgence of this infection in the UK not only in the ethnic minorities but also in the Caucasian population. Children show a high predisposition to developing extrapulmonary TB and its impact is greatest among infants and young children who tend to develop more severe extra-pulmonary disease, especially meningitis and miliary TB. HIV increases the risk of TBM and needs to be considered in these patients. Considering the resurgence of TB in the population, a strong index of suspicion needs to be maintained to enable early diagnosis and treatment.

Table 10.14.

CSF analysis	White cells/mm³	Protein (g/l)	Glucose (mmol/l)
Normal	<4 lymphocytes 0 polymorphs	<0.4	>2.2 (or ~2/3 plasma)
Acute bacterial meningitis	200-20 000 polymorphs	1-5	Usually low
Tuberculous meningitis	25-100, mainly lymphocytes except in early stages when mainly polymorphs	Usually 1-2 but may be much higher	Usually low
Cryptococcal meningitis	~50 (0-800) mainly lymphocytes	~1 (0.2-5)	Normally low, average 1.7
Viral meningitis	5- >1000, mainly lymphocytes except in early stages when mainly polymorphs	Usually <1, may be greater in severe cases	Normal but may be low in some cases of mumps and HSV1

CASE 10.15

A 5-year-old girl was admitted with a 5-day history of sore throat and increasing jaundice. She had not had abdominal pain or diarrhoea, but her urine was darker than usual, and her stool was "orange". Two weeks previously she had travelled to Florida and Egypt. Examination revealed a pale, but active, jaundiced child, with a temperature of 37°C, pink ears and throat, and no other abnormality noted. Her blood results are as follows:

Hb 5.4	Na 136
MCH 29	K 4.2
MCV 87.4	Urea 4.6
WCC 13.7	Creatinine 47
Platelets 96	Bilirubin 62
Direct Coombes' negative	
Antibody screen negative	
Protein 69	ALT 12
Albumin 42	ALP 174

Throat swab grew *Mycoplasma pneumoniae*. Infectious mononucleosis screen was negative and G6PD screen was normal.

a. Which of the following diagnoses is excluded by the above results?
SELECT *ONE* ANSWER ONLY
  i. Autoimmune haemolytic anaemia *(Mycoplasma)*
  ii. Viral hepatitis
  iii. Hereditary spherocytosis
  iv. G6PD deficiency

b. What further investigation would you do to help make a diagnosis?
SELECT *ONE* ANSWER ONLY
  i. GAL-1-PUT
  ii. Osmotic fragility test
  iii. CT scan abdomen
  iv. Stool for bacteriology
  v. Bone marrow aspirate

The next day the child became lethargic and was noted to be short of breath on exertion. Hb was 5.1. Decision was made to give a blood transfusion. After receiving 40 ml of blood, her temperature increased from 37.5°C to 38.5°C.

c. What is the most likely cause of the temperature?
SELECT *ONE* ANSWER ONLY
  i. Overheated blood
  ii. Sepsis
  iii. Transfusion reaction
  iv. Graft versus host disease
  v. Line infection

ANSWERS TO CASE 10.15

a. i. Autoimmune haemolytic anaemia *(Mycoplasma)*
b. ii. Osmotic fragility test
c. iii. Transfusion reaction

To help make a diagnosis other information required includes:
    recent drug history
    racial origin
    previous episodes of jaundice and past medical history
    family history of jaundice
    infectious diseases contact history
    ingestion of fava beans or broad beans
    hepatosplenomegaly

These blood results demonstrate a non-autoimmune haemolytic anaemia (HA) and thrombocytopaenia. Mycoplasma can cause a HA, but it is an autoimmune HA characterised by a positive direct Coombs, where antibody typically reacts with the red cells at 4°C (cold type); so this infection is not the cause of this anaemia. An osmotic fragility test is needed to exclude hereditary spherocytosis. There may be a family history as it is inherited as autosomal dominant, variable expression. The G6PD screen will need to be repeated when the child is better. G6PD is still a possible diagnosis despite the normal screen. G6PD levels may be normal during haemolytic episodes because of increased red cell turnover, so if normal, test again when acute haemolysis is over. If a diagnosis is made, treat with folic acid and give advice to avoid exacerbating factors (anti-malarials, paracetamol, penicillin, fava and broad beans). Siblings should be screened.

If a fever develops during a transfusion, the most likely diagnosis, and one that needs urgent management, is a transfusion reaction. Management of a transfusion reaction: stop transfusion; reassess; look for focus of infection; if none, consider a possible transfusion reaction; ensure the child is cardiovascularly stable, look for signs of shock (delayed cap refill time, tachycardia, and later hypotension), and treat. Check that the identity of the recipient is the same as that stated on the compatibility label and that this corresponds with the blood being transfused; send blood from the child, and the rest of the blood being transfused, to the laboratory for culture to exclude bacterial contamination. Also:

- repeat group and cross-match on pre- and post-transfusion samples
- do a direct Coombs on the post-transfusion sample to look for antibody on the red cell surface (if positive, this indicates a transfusion reaction; also positive with autoimmune HA, drug-induced HA, and haemolytic disease of the newborn)
- check plasma for haemoglobinaemia
- look for evidence of disseminated intravascular coagulation (clotting screen, increased fibrinogen, degradation products)
- examine urine for haemoglobinuria
- take further samples of blood several hours later to look for falling haemoglobin and rising bilirubin
- if no positive findings look at the patient's serum 5-10 days later for red or white cell antibodies

CASE 10.16

A 4-year-old boy presents with a 2-week history of fever, lethargy and an intermittent rash. On examination, he is clinically anaemic and has cervical lymphadenopathy, a warm effusion in the left knee and a macular, salmon-pink rash over his trunk. His temperature chart clearly shows twice-daily fevers that exceed 41°C and do not reduce with non-steroidal anti-inflammatory drugs (NSAIDs). The GP has reported his CRP level as being elevated at 115.

What are your differential diagnoses at this stage?

SELECT *TWO* ANSWERS ONLY

  i. Polyarteritis nodosa
  ii. Measles
  iii. Systemic-onset juvenile idiopathic arthritis
  iv. Acute lymphoblastic leukaemia
  v. Rheumatic fever
  vi. Kawasaki syndrome
  vii. Rubella

ANSWERS TO CASE 10.16

iii. Systemic-onset juvenile idiopathic arthritis
iv. Acute lymphoblastic leukaemia

Differential diagnoses at this stage should include systemic-onset juvenile idiopathic arthritis (JIA), infection and acute lymphoblastic leukaemia.

Systemic-onset JIA

The definition of a JIA is a chronic arthritis persisting for more than a minimum of 6 consecutive weeks in one or more joints. Systemic-onset JIA usually commences before the age of 5 years, although occasionally presents in older children and adults. It accounts for approximately 10% of children with JIA. The systemic features may precede arthritis by weeks or months. The features include a high spiking temperature (often twice daily, dipping below the baseline in between spikes), a classic rash that consists of discrete, salmon-pink macules that tend to be migratory and visceral involvement (including hepatosplenomegaly, lymphadenopathy and pericarditis). The children often appear acutely unwell. There may be a murmur heard on auscultation. Investigations which should be carried out initially include:

FBC and film
blood cultures
CXR
viral screen and autoimmune profile

Acute treatment of this child involves broad-spectrum antibiotics until the infection screen has been obtained, non-steroidal anti-inflammatory drugs (NSAIDs), and oral or i.v. steroids once infection has been excluded. Gentle, paced physiotherapy and nutritional support should be given if necessary.

Diagnosis of systemic-onset JIA is difficult initially, particularly in the absence of arthritis. It is important to exclude malignancy, sepsis, inflammatory bowel disease and vasculitides. Laboratory tests are helpful in exclusion of other entities but are not specific in systemic JIA. The course and duration of this disease is variable. The systemic features tend to subside during the initial months or years but may recur with flares of the arthritis. The arthritis may become aggressive, affecting many joints and occasionally necessitating their replacement.

Treatment is multidisciplinary. Medications include NSAIDs, prednisolone (i.v., pulsed, oral or intra-articular) and second-line therapy (methotrexate, cyclophosphamide and anti-tumour necrosis factor). Approximately 50% of children recover completely with no significant disability in adult life.

Table 10.17.1

		Biopsy		
		Positive	Negative	Total
Blood test	**Positive**	119	45	164
	Negative	26	460	486
	Total	145	505	650

A group of clinicians wished to use a blood test to screen for a certain condition. In order to determine the accuracy of this screening test, a comparison needed to be made with a definitive test such as a biopsy. Six hundred and fifty individuals were tested using both the blood test and the biopsy and the above results were obtained:

a. What is the specificity of the test?
   SELECT *ONE* ANSWER ONLY
   i. 119/145
   ii. 26/460
   iii. 460/486
   iv. 460-26/486

b. What is the negative predictive value for this test?
   SELECT *ONE* ANSWER ONLY
   i. 460/650
   ii. 26/460
   iii. 460/486
   iv. 460-26/486

a. i. 119/145
b. iii. 460/486

The prevalence is the proportion of subjects affected by the disease. The number that actually has the disease is identified by those with a positive result from the biopsy, i.e. 145.

Thus the prevalence of the disease is 145/650 = 0.223 or 22.3%.

The sensitivity measures how sensitive the screening test is for detecting the disease when it is actually present. The sensitivity for this test is 119/145 = 0.821 or 82.1%.

The specificity is the proportion of subjects that don't have the disease that are correctly identified by the screening test as not having it. Therefore, the specificity is 460/505 = 0.911 or 91.1%.

The positive predictive value is the proportion of subjects that have a positive test result that do have the disease. So the positive predictive value for this example is 119/164 = 0.726 or 72.6%.

The negative predictive value is the proportion of subjects that have a negative test result that don't actually have the disease. Therefore, the value will lie between 0 and 1. For this example, the negative predictive value is 460/486 = 0.947 or 94.7%.

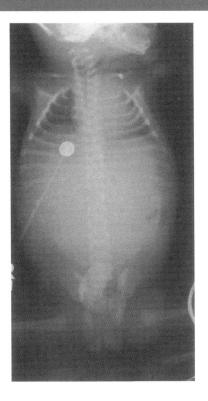

Fig 10.18

A neonate born at 26 weeks' gestation was intubated in the labour ward, given surfactant and ventilated. On day 2 the baby deteriorated, developing abdominal distension and increasing oxygen requirements. Abdominal radiograph suggested a GI perforation. After recovery it was difficult to establish feeds. Difficult i.v. access resulted in the insertion of a Broviac line into the right internal jugular vein. This was subsequently removed because of line infection. Two days later the baby collapsed. Arterial blood gas showed a pH of 7.0, pCO_2 9 kPa, pO_2 3 kPa, HCO_3 22 mmol/l and a base excess of −6 mmol/l. The CXR is shown.

a. What does the X-ray show?
SELECT *ONE* ANSWER ONLY
 i. Right-sided pneumothorax
 ii. Right-sided pleural effusion
 iii. Right-sided consolidation
 iv. Right-sided collapse

b. What is the most likely diagnosis?
SELECT *ONE* ANSWER ONLY
 i. Chylothorax
 ii. Pneumonia
 iii. Hyaline membrane disease
 iv. Pulmonary haemorrhage

ANSWERS TO CASE 10.18

a. ii. Right-sided pleural effusion
b. i. Chylothorax

Management entails an emergency thoracocentesis to relieve the pressure on the lung and improve the ventilation. Pleural fluid should be sent for microscopy, culture, electrolytes, triglycerides, and fat-laden macrophages.

With the history of the broviac line, the most likely diagnosis is a chylothorax associated with insertion of a central line.

Chylothoraces can also occur due to a congenital malformation of the thoracic duct (e.g. in Turner's syndrome) or secondary to trauma (e.g. after cardiac surgery).

Management of a chylothorax:
- Insert a chest drain or repeated thoracocentesis.
- Nutritional management is a major concern. An enteral diet rich in medium–chain triglycerides (MCTs) should be considered for a minimum period of 2 weeks. In theory, this allows the main fat content of the diet to be absorbed directly into the portal system, rather than being digested, absorbed across the brush border into the enterocyte, reassimilated and entering the lymphatic system. An alternative option is to keep the infant nil orally with total parenteral nutrition containing sufficient amounts of calories, protein, electrolytes, vitamins, etc. to compensate for losses. These infants often develop protein depletion and may require albumin infusions. They may also be immunocompromised on the basis of lymphocyte and immuno-globulin depletion.
- Infuse somatostatin analogue, which may reduce chyle drainage.
- When medical management fails, consider surgical ligation of the thoracic duct, pleurodesis or thoracoabdominal shunting.
- Careful counselling of parents regarding this complication is needed and the probable need for a prolonged period of intensive care. Mortality rates vary in the literature, but the majority survives.

CASE 10.19

A previously healthy 3-year-old child developed a cough for which she received no treatment. Ten days later she developed a puffy face and swollen ankles. Her parents reported a decreased appetite, but good fluid intake, and occasional abdominal pain. Examination revealed a well-hydrated, normotensive child with facial oedema. Her abdomen was distended with ascites but non-tender. She had pitting oedema to the thighs. Urinalysis showed protein ++++ and blood +. Her serum albumin was 3 g/l.

a. What other parameter is characteristically abnormal in this condition?
    SELECT THE *MOST APPROPRIATE* ANSWER
    i. Hb
    ii. C3
    iii. IgA
    iv. Platelets
    v. Cholesterol

b. Which renal lesion is the most common cause of this disease in childhood?
    SELECT *ONE* ANSWER ONLY
    i. Focal sclerosis
    ii. Minimal change nephropathy
    iii. IgA nephropathy
    iv. Goodpasture's syndrome
    v. Basement membrane disease

c. Which children with this condition need discussion with or referral to a paediatric nephrologist?
    SELECT *TWO* ANSWERS ONLY
    i. Proteinuria >1 week
    ii. Age >12 years
    iii. Hypertension
    iv. Serum albumin <2 g/l
    v. All children <5 years

ANSWERS TO CASE 10.19

a. v. Cholesterol
b. ii. Minimal change nephropathy
c. ii. Age >12 years
    iii. Hypertension

Nephrotic syndrome is a clinical condition resulting from the loss of large amounts of protein from the blood into the urine. This is associated with hypoproteinaemia, oedema, and hypercholesterolaemia, and lipiduria. Nephrotic-range proteinuria is found when there is 4+ protein on the urine dipstick, which correlates with proteinuria of more than 40 mg/kg/day.

The nephrotic syndrome may be a feature of any form of childhood glomerulonephritis or may be secondary to other systemic diseases, nephrotoxins or allergic reactions. In approximately 80% of children the aetiology is minimal change nephrotic syndrome. Of these, 60% are between the ages of 1 and 6. Older children are likely to have other underlying types of glomerulonephritis (i.e. not minimal change) and thus they often have a renal biopsy earlier in the course of the disease.

The concentration of plasma proteins is also decreased because of increased urinary losses, decreased synthesis, or increased catabolism, such as albumin, coagulation inhibitors and IgG. Some plasma proteins are, however, increased (possibly because of unregulated hepatic production in response to hypoalbuminaemia) such as coagulation factors, antifibrinolysins, and most lipoproteins. Cholesterol is also elevated in most cases.

Children with the following atypical features need discussion with or referral to a paediatric nephrologist:

● age <1 year or >12 years
● significant haematuria
● hypertension
● family history
● unexplained renal dysfunction

Any children who fail to respond to appropriate treatment with steroids or who have problems with steroid side-effects also need referral.

Index